S0-AGX-824

# Healing Touch
## A Guidebook for Practitioners
### 2nd Edition

# DEDICATION

To all those who seek healing for themselves and their relationships—and in so doing heal others for the highest good.

# Healing Touch
## A Guidebook for Practitioners
### 2nd Edition

**DOROTHEA HOVER-KRAMER, EdD, RN**
with contributing authors
**Janet Mentgen, BSN, RN**
**Norma Geddes, PhD, RN**
**Sharon Scandrett-Hibdon, PhD, RN**
**Victoria Slater, PhD, RN, CHTP/I, HNC**

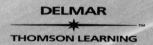
DELMAR
™
THOMSON LEARNING

Australia Canada Mexico Singapore Spain United Kingdom United States

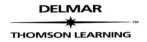

**DELMAR**

**THOMSON LEARNING** ™

Healing Touch: A Guidebook for Practitioners
by Dorothea Hover-Kramer, EdD, RN

**Business Unit Director:**
William Brottmiller

**Executive Marketing Manager:**
Dawn F. Gerrain

**Art/Design Coordinator:**
Robert S. Plante

**Product Developmental Manager:**
Marion Waldman

**Channel Manager:**
Gretta Oliver

**Cover Design:**
Robert S. Plante

**Product Development Editor:**
Jill Rembetski

**Project Editor:**
Maureen M.E. Grealish

**Editorial Assistant:**
Robin Irons

**Production Coordinator:**
Anne Sherman

COPYRIGHT © 2002 by Delmar,
a division of Thomson Learning, Inc. Thomson
Learning™ is a trademark used herein under license

Printed in the United States
7 8 9 10 XXX 09 08 07

For more information contact Delmar Thomson
Learning
3 Columbia Circle
PO Box 15015
Albany, NY 12212-5015.

Or find us on the World Wide Web at
http://www.delmar.com

ALL RIGHTS RESERVED. No part of this work cov-
ered by the copyright hereon may be reproduced or
used in any form or by any means—graphic, electronic, or mechanical, including photocopying,
recording, taping, Web distribution or information
storage and retrieval systems—without written permission of the publisher.

For permission to use material from this text or product, contact us by
Tel    (800) 730-2214
Fax   (800) 730-2215
www.thomsonrights.com

Library of Congress
Cataloging-in-Publication Data

Hover-Kramer, Dorothea
   Healing touch: guidebook for practitioners /
   Dorothea Hover-Kramer, with contributing
   authors Janet Mentgen ... [et al.]
     p. cm.
   Includes index
   ISBN-13: 978–0–7668–2519–2
   ISBN-10: 0–7668–2519–1 (alk. paper)
   1. Touch—Therapeutic use. I. Mentgen, Janet.
   II. Title.
   RZ999 .H67 2001
   615.8'52—dc21
                                            2001042337

## NOTICE TO THE READER

Publisher does not warrant or guarantee any of the products described herein or perform any independent analysis in connection with any of the product information contained herein. Publisher does not assume, and expressly disclaims, any obligation to obtain and include information other than that provided to it by the manufactur-
er.

The reader is expressly warned to consider and adopt all safety precautions that might be indicated by the activities herein and to avoid all potential hazards. By following the instructions contained herein, the reader willing-
ly assumes all risks in connection with such instructions.

The Publisher makes no representation or warranties of any kind, including but not limited to, the warranties of
fitness for particular purpose or merchantability, nor are any such representations implied with respect to the
material set forth herein, and the publisher takes no responsibility with respect to such material. The publisher
shall not be liable for any special, consequential, or exemplary damages resulting, in whole or part, from the readers' use of, or reliance upon, this material.

# INTRODUCTION TO THE HEALER SERIES

*Lynn Keegan, PhD, RN, Series Editor*
*Director, Holistic Health Consultants*
*Port Angeles, Washington*

*M*ost health care professionals care for others with compassion; they begin their formal education with this ideal. Many retain this orientation after graduation, and some manage their entire careers under this guiding principle of caring. Many of us, however, tend to forget this ideal in the hectic pace of our professional and personal lives. We may become discouraged and feel a sense of burnout.

I have spoken at hundreds of conferences with thousands of caregivers. Their experience of frustration and failure is quite common. These professionals feel themselves spread as pawns across a health care system too large to control or understand. In part, this may be because they have forgotten their true roles as healers.

When individuals redirect their personal vision and empower themselves, an entire pattern may begin to change. And so it is now with the health care profession. Most of us conceptualize our roles as much more than a vocation. We are greater than our individual roles as scientists, specialists, or care deliverers. We currently search for a name to put on our new conception of the empowered caregiver. The recently introduced term *healer* aptly describes the qualities of an increasing number of clinicians, educators, administrators, and practitioners. Today most caregivers are awakening to the realization that they have the potential for healing.

It is my feeling that most, when awakened and guided to develop their own healing potential, will function as healers. Thus, the concept of caregiver as healer is born. When we realize we have the ability to evoke others' healing, as well as care for them, a shift of consciousness begins to occur. As individual awareness and changes in skill building occur, a collective understanding of this new concept emerges. This knowledge, along with a shift in attitudes and new kinds of behavior, allows empowered caregivers to renew themselves in an expanded role. The Healer Series is born out of the belief that caregivers are ready to embrace guidance that inspires them in their journeys of empowerment. Each book in the series may stand alone or be used in complementary fashion with other books. I hope and believe that information herein will strengthen you both personally and professionally, and provide you with the help and confidence to embark upon the path of a healer.

*Titles in the Healer Series:*

**Healing with Complementary and Alternative Therapies**

**Healing Touch: A Guidebook for Practitioners, 2nd Edition**

**Healing Life's Crises: A Guide for Nurses**

**The Nurse's Meditative Journal**

**Healing Nutrition**

**Healing the Dying, 2nd Edition**

**Awareness in Healing**

**Creative Imagery**

**Profiles of Nurse Healers**

**Healing Addictions**

**Healing and the Grief Process**

**Spirituality: Living our Connectedness**

# CONTENTS

## SECTION V
## SELF-CARE OF THE PRACTITIONER

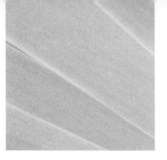

# Introduction

*h*istorically, late in the 1970s, an explosion of interest in new approaches to health care emerged. In psychotherapy there was the advent of self-help programs, support groups, learning for personal growth, and self-awareness — the human potential movement as it came to be called. People no longer had to be mentally ill to want more out of life and to gain self-understanding. Getting help for a life crisis or transition became normal and acceptable. Better yet, people found that early intervention with physical or emotional needs prevented further deterioration or onset of chronic conditions.

In the 1980s this trend toward early intervention and increased self-care led to growing public interest in treatment modalities that went beyond usual medical approaches. In psychotherapy a variety of training programs in communication skills, interpersonal relationships, encounter groups, and the transpersonal dimension emerged. For care of the physical body a variety of alternatives gained public recognition, leading to mainstream acknowledgment of massage, chiropractic, acupuncture, and biofeedback. The formation of the American Holistic Nurses' Association (AHNA) and the American Holistic Medical Association (AHMA) in the early 1980s was inevitable on the crest of this wave.

In the 1990s the social and legal acceptance of these new modalities became a major focus, with emphasis on health care reform, streamlining complex health care administration, and cost containment. New information about the complex interrelationship between the mind and the body has become available as well. Because of their effectiveness in preventing further disability, some unique approaches focusing on this interconnectedness have set a new standard of care. For example, Dr. Dean Ornish's programs of stress management and imagery for persons diagnosed with cardiac symptoms is reimbursed by third party payers to assist in preventing the need for cardiac bypass surgery.

In the 21st century this background of public interest in other ways of managing health care has encouraged approaches based on the human energy system and how it can be enhanced for healing. Healing Touch, as presented in this book, is an example of such an approach. It is best understood as a complement or adjunct to other ways of treating the body/mind interconnection. Caregiving with Healing Touch involves internal preparation of the helping professional and specific techniques based on knowledge and skill. To further round out the picture, the history, research, and operating theoretical framework are presented with numerous applications and case examples. Beyond the basic understanding, however, no equipment is needed, allowing a welcome diversion for practitioners from high-tech medical practice. The caregiver works with intuition, skill, a compassionate heart, and sensitive hands.

The energetic approaches, of which Healing Touch and Therapeutic Touch are best known in the health care field, have received increasing public interest and support. Many hospitals, nationally and internationally, have policies that allow skilled practitioners of either modality to implement an energetic approach when appropriate. Health care consumers are requesting this work before and after surgery and in emergency and intensive care settings.

On a more personal note, my professional development as an adult closely parallels this historical framework. In the 1970s, I was an enthusiastic consumer of the human potential movement and its many therapies. In the next decade, I joined the American Holistic Nurses' Association (AHNA) and served on its board for seven years, helping to foster and encourage the now well-established holistic nursing program and the Healing Touch program as AHNA's Education Chair. As the groundbreaking work in Healing Touch progressed, I became one of the first certified practitioners and certified instructors (#002 on both counts, after Healing Touch prinicipal founder Janet Mentgen). Forever unforgettable will be the thousands of wide-eyed students that filled those early classes with their questions, their curiosity, and their willingness to learn what was then a very new paradigm. Equally memorable is the wonderful group of dedicated, pioneering early practitioners and teachers, many of whom are now leaders in the ever-growing field of Healing Touch, as the reader will see in this volume.

My own journey has expanded in new directions this past five years toward utilizing energy healing concepts in my work as a health psychologist, in developing courses for counselors and therapists, and in helping to co-found the Association of Comprehensive Energy Psychology in 1999, which now has over 500 members worldwide. In all likelihood, the 21st century will see a vast expansion of energetic modalities in all aspects of health care. The direction of the future is evident in the growing public interest in complementary therapies and alternate ways of not only treating illness but also in achieving and maintaining high levels of well-being.

The roots of this intense personal interest in healing and all its implications lie in my wounded past. Growing up as a young child in war-torn Berlin, Germany, there seemed to be little hope for living and wellness, other than through a faith in some form of divine guidance. My intuition served me well in finding the people who had "light" around them and could assist a motherless child. I learned to be rather objective about deaths in my family and those around me, as all of the events were clearly beyond my feeble understanding. I often nursed injured animals, and took in rejected or broken dolls. I especially remember passing my hands slowly and purposely over injured birds that neighbors brought me. Since many of the fledglings were likely to die in spite of my food, water, and hand-directed efforts, I decided to pray that they go in the direction that would serve their highest good, whether that be death or life. If they passed on, my sister and I would hold elaborate funerals in the backyard, a very appropriate, and probably therapeutic activity for those disrupted times. If the little birds lived, my heart would rejoice in a different way. In these simple acts lay the seeds of work with animals and people, connections and ideas, that would nourish a lifetime.

I never forgot those little animals or the sense of satisfaction of knowing that I could do something to help. When I entered nursing school I wondered when we would learn more about such healing, as I was convinced that this was in the spirit of Florence Nightingale's ideas about nursing and caregiving. Alas, nursing in the 1960s tried its best to be objective rather than spiritual—giving injections, following orders, and charting were our prescribed domains. When I asked my professors about healing they looked puzzled. The answers were to come much more slowly as new potentials opened within nursing and all health care professions in the succeeding decades.

This volume is the second edition of what has become a classic textbook, *Healing Touch: A Resource for Healthcare Professionals* (1996) within the Nurse as Healer series at Delmar. In a short ten years Healing Touch has "come of age," developing its own organizational, certification, and research structures along with many fascinating courses for further development of the practitioner. This revised, expanded version reflects and celebrates the tremendous growth in both the depth and breadth of the program. It is much more now than just another resource for health care professionals, and, since there will be many other books about Healing Touch and various related programs on the market, we have chosen to call it *Healing Touch: Guidebook for Practitioners*, emphasizing this work's role as the basic textbook for novice or experienced readers.

My thanks go to the many, both named and unnamed, whose vision carried the program forward in the last ten years, to all those whose open hearts and spirits permitted healing ideas to nourish themselves and those in their care. To Lynn Keegan, longtime friend and colleague, go deep thanks for holding the vision for and empowering the Nurse as Healer series. To the folks at Delmar, notably Jill Rembetski, a special appreciation.

Specifically, I want to thank each of the contributing authors for their extraordinary chapter contributions. First, of course, is Janet Mentgen, official Healing Touch founder, whose direct, no nonsense style of helping clients and teaching students captured all of our imaginations. In addition, she supervises the ongoing administration of Healing Touch worldwide. Her chapters 9–12 identify and describe most of the Healing Touch techniques as they are currently taught; her contributions to the first chapter are in keeping track of the history and development of the program. Sharon Scandrett-Hibdon is a long-time contributor to

Healing Touch, and in this volume she gives sensitive cross-cultural understanding to our notions of healing. In addition, she describes the exciting new programs and specialty areas that have developed mostly since the original text was published. Norma Geddes is a nursing researcher whose special gifts include understanding both quantitative and qualitative research and showing examples of fine qualitative Healing Touch research in the third chapter. It is fascinating to share in her observations of personal transformation in Healing Touch practitioners. And last but not least, my appreciation goes to Vicki Slater, whose love of knowledge permeates every page of the chapter exploring the scientific basis of Healing Touch. Her work offers a new and delicious feast for the mind.

The author would also like to acknowledge the following reviewers:

Elizabeth Schaeffer Teichler, RN-C, FNP, HNC, PhD (c)
School of Nursing
University of Colorado Health Sciences Center
Louisville, CO

Kathleen Palladino, BS, RN
Angel Hill Wellness Center
Spencertown, NY

Karilee H. Shames, PhD, RN, HNC
College of Nursing
Florida Atlantic University
Fort Lauderdale, FL

Hopefully, from me as the author and compiler of this revised volume, the reader will gain a sense of the scope of current practice of Healing Touch. There are hundreds of updates and new references, but, more importantly, the language is clearer and more precise as we have had time to season and grow. Lastly, I invite the reader to share in some of the excitement about energy healing concepts and their practical applications in many professional as well as personal settings.

As all healing is ultimately self-healing, I invite you to join me in a special adventure—that of discovering the healer within.

Dorothea Hover-Kramer,
Clinical Director, Behavioral Health Consultants
Poway, CA

# How To Use This Book

*t*his book is intended to be the current, basic textbook about the concepts and techniques of Healing Touch (HT). It is a primer for anyone who is curious about HT and wants to understand its practice. For students who are taking HT classes it serves as an in-depth resource, in addition to the illustrated workbooks distributed in the classrooms. As there are many books being written about specialty areas within the advanced practice of HT, no attempt is made here to cover all the details but rather to give you, the reader (and potential healing practitioner), the essential framework from which HT operates and to identify many of the resources for ongoing reading and information.

A quick perusal of the table of contents may help you to identify your most burning questions and to start with the section that is most helpful. Some of you will seek a good theory and research base to accept the applications for practice that we suggest. Others may want to have a grasp of the HT techniques before learning the underlying concepts, such as presented in the chapters about the human energy system. The book is intended to meet you where you are in your own stage of development. With this in mind, you may enjoy reading Section V, Self-Care of the Practitioner, before exploring information about the HT program in Sections I and III.

Each chapter has a number of references listed at the end that relate to the body of the text and may also lead you into interesting further exploration of energy healing concepts.

The index gives a quick reference for application of HT concepts to specific human needs. As in the previous edition, this feature may be the one that practitioners find most useful in daily practice. The index also allows access to the writing of leading theorists and topical information.

In addition, we have provided a glossary of terms most used in this second edition, sample documentations of HT assessments and interventions, a sample informed consent document for use with clients, as well as information about the HT certification process, and resources for information about the many national and international classes.

One of the significant contributions of Healing Touch is that it integrates easily with other modalities the practitioner may already be using: the many body-oriented therapies, traditional medical practice in hospital and clinical settings, and established practices of psychotherapy. In Section IV we also explore the bridges with medical settings, many of which are constantly developing as physicians and nurses utilize energy concepts as a complement to the work they are currently doing.

Certainly, all healing work must begin with the practitioner's own healing. Although a perfect state of mental and physical health is an unrealistic expectation, a sense of direction or movement toward increasing wellness is essential. Because we as healers are role models through our relative wellness, we must begin by "walking our talk" — thinking, breathing, living, doing, and being — in a holistic way. This means that we respect the physical body and its needs, learn to release emotional tension, clear the mind of clutter, and connect with our spiritual essence on a daily basis.

In the last chapter we summarize the adventure of exploring the world of HT by looking again at the beginning. In the last ten years, the HT program has grown phenomenally in size and stature, to become a recognized and established entity in the health care field. As we consider the future, we foresee a growing acceptance of energy-based modalities to augment many traditional and complementary forms of physical and emotional healing. We will each be a part of this unfolding adventure. Enjoy the journey!

# History, Research, and Background of Healing Touch

*In this first section we explore the development of Healing Touch (HT) as a major force among the many energy-oriented healing modalities. This includes an overview of significant developments in HT since its inception, leading to the steady growth of the program nationally and internationally. We explore concepts of healing in human history that support the emergence of energetic modalities, and specific research that describes the outcomes of HT interventions. In addition, we consider some of the scientific background that helps us to understand the impact of HT on both its clients and practitioners.*

# The Development of Healing Touch as a Major Force in Energy-Oriented Healing Practices

*Janet Mentgen, BS, RN and Dorothea Hover-Kramer, EdD, RN*

> *"Healing is the ongoing movement toward health, harmony, and wholeness."*
>
> —Dorothea Hover-Kramer

## TEN YEAR CELEBRATION: HEALING TOUCH INTERNATIONAL CONFERENCE, 2000

There are many milestones in the fascinating development of HT, a course and program that was designed to help nurses and caregivers to assist those in need. One of the most recent milestones was the vibrant success of the fifth HT International Conference, with over 500 participants attending in the lush mountains of Kauai, that celebrated the tenth anniversary of HT as a major force for healing among health care professionals and laypersons.

As participants assembled from all over the world, Janet Mentgen, founder and ongoing director of the Colorado Center for HT, noted that there are now 1,020 certified HT practitioners and 146 certified HT instructors, and that over the previous ten years, a total of 3,801 workshops have been given in the United States to over 54,867 participants. Courses are also held in Australia, New Zealand, Canada, Netherlands, Germany, Finland, Great Britain, South Africa, Trinidad, Peru, Nicaragua. Beyond the statistics, however, there was the warmth and sense of inherent goodwill that was palpable to all at the conference.

What allowed for such rapid expansion of a simple healing modality to a worldwide audience? Was there an unusual constellation of events and people that brought this program to such a dramatic focus? Or, was it simply an idea whose time had come?

## BEGINNINGS OF HT AND DIFFERENTIATION FROM OTHER ENERGY HEALING MODALITIES

In the past thirty years, perhaps in response to the highly technological medical system, a number of courses and programs have been developed to explore broad concepts of healing through awareness of the human energy system. Some have developed around the teachings of such specific healers as Barbara Brennan, Brugh Joy, and Rosalyn Bruyere, while others have presented a philosophy for approaching human distress via modern interpretations of ancient healing practices. Best known among the healing philosophies is Therapeutic Touch, a well-documented and often researched intervention, founded over thirty years ago by Dr. Dolores Krieger and Dora Kunz. Other approaches, such as pranic healing and shamanic practices are implemented by practitioners worldwide in various cultures and contexts.

From the beginning, HT was envisioned as a specific program of study to teach an identifiable curriculum for learner development and to support and recognize its practitioners in their unfolding as energy healers. Because the specific course design incorporated the teachings of many well-known healers as well as concepts from shamanic and aborigine traditions, the name "Healing Touch" seemed to best match the vision of the three nurses who met on May 1, 1989 to determine what to call the new program. They were Janet Mentgen, who had been teaching healing classes for several years in the Denver area, Susan Morales, now coordinator of the Canadian HT offices, and the author of this book. Later that year, a task force consisting of Janet, Sharon Scandrett-Hibdon, Myra Till-Tovey, and the author began defining the program more clearly and suggested integration of the course material as a continuing education offering through the American Holistic Nurses' Association. The first classes were taught at the end of 1989, and from then on, all those who were willing learned and taught actively to give HT its phenomenal start and visibility.

## EVOLUTION OF THE HT COURSE

Because Janet had a good working knowledge of the skills needed for successful healing practice, the five part course outline, building from beginning to advanced levels, fell into place easily as a curriculum pathway. More challenging was the art of giving language to traditions that had often simply been passed from one generation to another and conceptualizing the work within the framework of modern health care knowledge. Many writers, teachers, and students were prime movers in developing this new language. But, the development of the entire program from its humble beginnings to the current level of influence was the tireless work of many—the dedicated, generous nurses who attended classes when we only had flimsy hand-outs; the non-nurse participants who added their curiosity about how body, mind, and spirit interact; the leadership council of AHNA who encouraged and enhanced the program objectives until 1996; the untiring office staff at the central office of the Colorado Center for  HT who coped with ever increasing public interest and demands; the hundreds of workshop organizers who believed that their friends would benefit from attending the classes and publicized the work; the teachers who held the vision of a health care system that would integrate both "high tech" and "high touch;" the many writers who are now publishing articles, workbooks, and books about specific aspects of HT; the HT newsletter editors and publishers who unite HT practitioners in their individual communities four times a year. We could go on and on as we begin to see the foundation of a well-established continuing education course that supported the development of a strong organization to advocate for and sustain its practitioners.

# EVOLUTION OF HT ORGANIZATION AND CERTIFICATION

Healing Touch has been defined since its beginnings as a program of study of various energy-linked healing approaches, including the many full body  and more localized techniques described in later chapters, which provides multidimensional healing to restore balance in the dynamic human being. In addition, HT is a program that recognizes practitioners who have completed the course of study and committed to their ongoing personal development. Since its inception, the HT organization has held the goal of acknowledging practitioners through certification. It was a fortuitous choice as, until this time, there was no way of recognizing or credentialling the large and growing body of energy healing practitioners.

The certification process began in essence with the very first HT course, with its well-defined objectives and learner outcomes, and culminated in the more formal dissemination of criteria for certification in 1993 and the setting up of the Certification Board. Initially, certification was awarded through the American Holistic Nurses' Association, with Dr. Ruth Johnston, Millie Freel, and the author as the first members of the HT Certification Board. In 1996, AHNA decided to limit its credentialling to their holistic nursing program, and Healing Touch International, Inc., a non-profit corporation, was established as a vehicle for HT certification. Since that time, there has been an executive administrator, who functions with a board of directors, and the hard-working Certification Board. (Details about certification and resources related to HT are located in Appendix B.)

Continued growth of the organization has come through the dedicated efforts of many small, regional support groups, who encourage ongoing practice of the techniques and discussion of issues. All those attending even a single HT class are eligible to attend  support groups to practice on other members as well as to receive HT interventions. Networking information for persons seeking an HT practitioner in their area is maintained through the central office, at the Colorado Center for HT.

The research arm of HT was established in 1994 with the leadership of Dr. Cynthia Hutchinson, and continues to grow as HT practitioners identify their scope of practice and the results of their interventions. An overview of this work is itemized in Chapter 3 of this work, showing how practitioners respond to the open-ended nature of healing work.

Another way that the organization has grown with the needs and interests of its members is that it now provides numerous courses in such HT specialty areas as working with animals, developing therapeutic communication skills, and exploring the spiritual aspects of healing. A description of these courses is given in Chapter 16, citing new developments for expanding practitioner resources.

## EMPHASIS ON PRACTITIONER DEVELOPMENT

Since the early beginnings of the HT program, there has been a profound emphasis on development of the healing practitioner. Client outcomes of increased relaxation, pain relief, and sense of well-being may vary somewhat depending on the needs and issues of the client; however, the communication between practitioner and client needs to be clear and free of attachment to any specific outcomes. This requires self-awareness and insight on the part of the healer. Centering, or focusing of one's intent for the highest good of the client, is the healer's primary resource for such objective clarity.

Throughout this book and in the HT classes, the theme of personal development and growth of the practitioner is reiterated. We have found that this emphasis not only enhances the client outcomes of relief from pain and distress but also changes the lives of the practitioner in profound ways. It is this personal development of practitioners and their colleagues that enriches the many circles and communities impacted by the HT modality.

## SUMMARY

We can conclude that HT as a movement has contributed significantly to increased well-being on a national and international scale. In reaching over

60,000 workshop participants in this country alone, HT has invited profession-als and laypersons alike to expand their potential for helping others as well as to become personally more focused and centered. In the succeeding chapters we will explore the theoretical basis for HT and related energy-oriented interventions along with techniques and applications in clinical settings. First, though, we want to explore the nature of healing, giving the historical context of this work, and to describe its emerging theoretical and research base.

# CHAPTER 2

# Concepts of Healing in Human History

*Sharon Scandrett-Hibdon, PhD, RN and*
*Dorothea Hover-Kramer, EdD, RN*

> *"Healing means moving into harmony within oneself, into wholeness in all aspects of one's being."*
>
> —Sharon Scandrett-Hibdon

## DEFINITIONS OF HEALING

The healing archetype has become increasingly visible and active in the late 20th and early 21st centuries at a time when medical technology has advanced to unprecedented heights. This seeming paradox can best be understood if we look at the inherent nature of healing as a creative, ongoing process that leads to increasing wholeness and harmony within each person. Beyond simply receiving a chemical or technological intervention when we are ill, we human beings seem to need a personal touch, a caring advocate, a belief that we can be restored to health, and a sense of hope and purpose in order to improve our sense of well-being.

There are many definitions of healing that encompass these qualities. *Merriam-Webster's Collegiate Dictionary* defines healing primarily as "the act of making sound or whole," whereas "to cause an undesirable condition to be overcome or mended" is secondary. The word *heal* is derived from the Greek stem *holos* and the Old English *haelen,* again implying wholeness and heartiness that goes beyond merely overcoming an illness.

Some theorists see life as a continuous flow of the essential life force or *Qi.* In this context, healing implies movement from a disturbed or complex flow pattern to a more harmonious one. This harmony encompasses our internal states as well as our relationships with the rest of the environment, our families, our communities, the world. Thus, the process of healing is conceptualized as an integral part of a functioning organic whole. Noted nursing theorist Martha

Rogers (described in Barrett, 1990) views healing as a movement toward harmony of the human and his environment to ever more evolved patterns of integration. Another nursing leader, Janet Quinn  (1992), describes healing as finding the right relationship between the individual and the entire environment. These definitions suggest that healing is not only an internal process but also one of harmonious interaction with our living environments.

Inherent in the concept of healing is a wider interpretation of our human reality: illness is not only a physical problem but an indication that there may be imbalance in other aspects of one's life as well. True well-being is much more than mere homeostasis in the organs. It is a harmonious evolution within physical, emotional, mental, and spiritual aspects of our being. While we are physical beings with material bodies, we are also emotional beings whose feelings can deeply influence the physical; we are mental, idea-generating beings whose thought patterns do indeed impact the physical and emotional aspects; and most importantly we are spiritual beings having a brief human experience who are ultimately connected to the Creative Source. Healing, in this light, is a multidimensional process toward ever-increasing levels of wellness in every part of our reality, and can occur even in the face of an ongoing or chronic physical problem.

# DIFFERENTIATION BETWEEN HEALING AND CURING

As we move forward in the 21st century, our definitions of illness and wellness are gradually changing. Until very recently, health was defined merely as the absence of physical distress or symptoms. With the evolution of a more integrative, holistic view, health is coming to be seen as ever-increasing levels of well-being, especially in the psychological and spiritual domains. Even aging is no longer seen as the inevitable demise of our physical prowess, but rather as an opportunity for learning more about our dynamic human systems to achieve and maintain high levels of functioning as we become more chronologically gifted. The presence of pain or *disease* is coming to be seen as a feedback signal from the entire human system that allows the individual to learn more about himself, not just something to be discarded or ignored.

In the current Western model of medical care, the goal is symptom removal or *cure*. While cure is defined in the dictionary as "something which corrects, heals or alleviates a harmful or troublesome situation" and is derived from the Latin word *cura*, for the care of souls, there is little in current, mainstream health care that addresses healing or care of the soul. If the goal of health is merely to be physically symptom free, then the giving of a chemical to remove pain, or surgery to remove a cancerous tumor, is all that is required. Curing, then, in current usage of the term, is quite different philosophically speaking from healing. Curing is seen as an external mechanism of providing physical symptom relief, preferably with complete eradication of the problem. Healing is seen as a multidimensional, ongoing process of movement toward wholeness, balance, and harmony from within the client. Curing in its current model is severely limited when there is an ongoing physical problem or life-threatening illness. Physicians or traditional caregivers will often say discouragingly to such patients, "We have done all we can." Healing, in contrast, is open-ended and allows the health care practitioner to explore the many possibilities for emotional, mental, and spiritual balancing even in the face of chronic or terminal physical illness. It is essentially hopeful and trusting of the innate healing capacity of the individual (see table 2.1).

This book focuses primarily on Healing Touch and the healing interventions that address rebalancing, or repatterning, to assist movement to higher levels of human functioning in all possible dimensions. It utilizes interventions that incorporate concepts of the human energy system. These interventions are natural and have been used, as we shall see, throughout human history. They promote a balancing of energy within the whole person, allowing, balance, harmony, and right relationship to emerge. Focused caring and touch from the caregiver appear to assist the client to relax, which permits the innate self-regulating mechanisms of the body to emerge. The practitioner aligns his energy and intention with the unlimited supply of Universal Energy to facilitate the client's personal evolution toward wholeness.

The movement toward healing in the client always comes from within but is facilitated by the intention and centering of the healer. We will explore the theoretical basis of these concepts and their application in the sections to come. For now, let us consider actual documentations of energy-oriented healing in human history and our understanding of endogenous healing as one model for our expanding view.

## DOCUMENTATIONS OF ENERGY HEALING

The term "energy healing" refers to a family of approaches to healing that are oriented to the condition of the human energy system. Inherent in all of them is assessment of the condition of the flow of energy via intuitive means of the various aspects of the biofield, the chakras, or the meridians, which will be described in detail later on. Interventions are directed to remove blockage of the flow of energy or *Qi* and to allow rebalancing of the system to occur.

A remarkable recent find allowed the world community to learn about the actual day to day life of a shepherd in the Italian Alps 5,200 years ago (PBS TV documentary *The Iceman* aired 2/27/2000). Because his body and skin were unusually well preserved, we even know what Iceman Oetzi had for dinner before he was frozen in time in a glacier. We know that he carried medicinal herbs including an antibiotic fungus, along with a special tinder box giving him numerous ways to start a fire. The clearly etched tattoo markings along his spine, and

| TABLE 2.1 | Comparison of Healing and Curing | |
|---|---|---|
| **Key Concepts** | **Healing** | **Curing** |
| Stem Word | *holos*–to make whole, to bring to balance | *cura*–care of souls |
| Current Meaning | movement to highest functional level possible, evolution toward increasing sense of well-being | to bring about recovery or release from a disease |
| Dimensions for Intervention | all aspects of the human being–physical, emotional, mental, and spiritual | predominantly the physical |
| Methods of Intervention | numerous complementary approaches that include nutritional care, body work, psychotherapy, prayer, energy-oriented approaches that balance the human energy system | mechanical–manipulation or removal of a diseased body part; chemical–administration of medication or chemotherapy |
| Desired Outcome | new insight and learning, about the *dis-ease* within each person, increased personal awareness | removal of symptoms; treatment ends when problem is alleviated |
| View of Illness | feeback for ongoing learning | external factors seen as causative agent |
| Role of Practitioner | practitioner works in open-ended partnership with client, mutual development of treatment goals and plan | skilled specialist who directs the curing protocol |

his right knee and foot were a total mystery. Further investigation showed that Oetzi suffered from osteoarthritis in these areas, but the tattoos made no sense until a practitioner of acupuncture examined the markings. They were lines tracing the specific meridians and acupoints, the electromagnetic pathways for the flow of *Qi* that would assist in relieving pain and facilitating healing in the affected areas. Stimulation of these acupoints by tattooing, heating, tapping, or insertion of needles continues to this day as the practice of acupuncture or acupressure and is one of many recognized energy healing modalities.

The significance of this discovery predates the known practice of acupuncture as a healing modality by several thousand years. Other energetic healing modalities are also in evidence through many cave drawings and the vast number of depictions from ancient cultures. Notable among these are healing dances practiced by bushmen and recorded in the rock art from Drakensberg Mountains in South Africa, believed to be several thousand years old (Katz, Biesele, and St. Denis, 1997). In cave drawings from France paintings of hands were inscribed, and healing with the hands is also recorded in early scriptures of all faiths (Harpur, 1994). The earliest Eastern written evidence of energetic healing is in the *Huang Ti Ching Su Wen* of 2500–5000 years ago (Veth, 1949). Pictures of healing from the Egyptian Third Dynasty demonstrate energetic conceptualization (Pavek, 1993), and Hover-Kramer (1993) reports numerous wall sculptures depicting the *ka*, the energetic envelope surrounding the physical body, in Egypt while working with an interpreter of the hieroglyphs.

## Early Energetic Names and Labels

In classical Greece, Hipprocrates used various words for energy as a force of flow from people's hands. Pythagoras, in the Greece of 500 BC, referred to vital energy perceived as a luminous body that could produce cures. Paracelsus referred to vital force and matter, calling it illiaster (Brennan, 1993, p.16). Throughout human history a variety of terms have been used by many cultures to name the vital life force, or energy, that resides in each living organism and differentiates the alive from the nonliving.

Table 2.2 suggests the universality of energy concepts in human cultures.

# BELIEFS ABOUT ILLNESS AND HEALING

In some ancient African beliefs, sickness or injury was understood as a process in which the individual was out of alignment with the animal spirits, ancestral dead, or deities (Katz, et al.,1997). The community of healers worked through healing dances to vigorously move energy (called *nlom*) through the patient's body in order to enhance his consciousness, to help him to see clearly into the problem, and to keep the patient from being carried off into the realm of death. These ritual dances were depicted in rock pictures in South Africa with lines of energy linking healers, animals, and humans. Transformation was the major goal and included a sense of harmony, equality, and spiritual connection.

In shamanism, the medicine man or woman traveled between the worlds to bring information to the people, to retrieve soul parts, to negotiate healing for the ill person, and to influence nature to assist the tribe (Villodo, 2000). Much power was imbued in these healers who knew the invisible spiritual world and interpreted environmental events, animal movement, and illness. Healing ritual, use of

| TABLE 2.2 | Some Equivalent Terms for Describing Human Energies |
|---|---|

| Energetic Name | Cultural Source |
|---|---|
| Apu | Incan heritage, Peru |
| Ankh | Ancient Egypt |
| Arunquiltha | Australian Aborigine |
| Bioenergy | USA/England |
| Biomagnetism | USA/England |
| Gana | South America |
| Huaca | Peru/Bolivia |
| Ki | Japan |
| Vital Life Force | General Usage |
| Mana | Polynesia |
| Orenda | Iroquois native Americans |
| Pneuma | Ancient Greece |
| Pran | India |
| Qi (pronounced "chee") | China |
| Subtle Energy | USA/Europe |
| Ton | Dakota native Americans |
| Walkan | Lakota native Americans |

herbs or concoctions, massage, intercession and interpretation were all important tools used by the shamans (Kharitidi, 1996; Guttenberg, 1997; Plotkin, 1993).

In the Orient, ancient practices worked with the flow of the sacred energy, called *Qi.* "*T'ai Qi*" and "*Qi Gong*" are two practices known in the West that help to move the vital life force for health maintenance as well as for healing of illness (Harpur, 1994). Acupuncture, an increasingly well-known health promoting modality, stimulates the movement of *Qi* along energy pathways, known as *meridians*, and is believed to balance the energy flows and blocked, or stagnant energy.

Another Eastern practice, known for 5,000 years, is the Ayurvedic tradition within yoga (Rose & Keegan, 2000). In this tradition, activation of the human energy vortices is used to balance the individual's basic constitution for self-healing and maintaining of balance.

In Western tradition, stories from the Hebrews who lived thousands of years ago held that obedience to the law and nation, through their covenant with God, were linked to physical health. The sins of one person were believed to create punishment for the whole nation via pestilence or plagues (Smith, 2000). Once again, we see the idea that being out of favor with God, being out of harmony with natural law, puts one at risk for becoming ill.

Holism was mentioned in early Greek culture in the schools of Aesculpius and Hippocrates, which became the foundations of modern medicine. Temples for healing with music, color, and dream incubation were a vital part of Greek culture.

In the Judeo-Christian tradition, Jesus gave many healings to drive out demonic forces and offered messages of hope to all. Forty-one incidents of Jesus' healing activity are recorded in the New Testament, and half involved touching, even of "untouchables" such as lepers (Smith, 2000). Christian healers are reported to have continued these compassionate acts even when they were later forbidden to do so by the powerful church establishment of the Middle Ages.

## THE USE OF ELECTROMAGNETICS

There is also a biomedical and electromagnetic history in physics that supports energetic healing. In the nineteenth century, Mesmer, Liebnitz, and Reichenbach cited aspects of electromagnetic field phenomena such as the attraction and repulsion of magnets to each other (Brennan, 1993). In the early 20th century, Kilner observed the human aura using colored screens and filters to see three layers. He also correlated auric configurations and disease states. Emanations from the auric field were detected by George de la Warr in the 1940s through radionic instruments. These instruments were used for diagnosis and distance healing. Wilhelm Reich in 1930 to 1950 developed a model of psychotherapy utilizing the human energy field. Later, Burr and Northrup observed the life field that demonstrates organization of the human energy field and developed the concept of circadian rhythms. They found that measurements of the energy field of seeds correlated with the strength or weakness of plants and that weakness of the life field of animals predated disease. This work was furthered by Ravitz in the 1950s, who observed thought fields that interfered with the life field to produce psychosomatic symptoms (all the preceding cited in Brennan, 1993, pp. 16–17).

In the 1960s, Bernard Grad attempted to demonstrate separation of energy transfer from psychic ability. It was his concept that healing went beyond belief and charisma. He studied three groups of people including healers, a control group, and depressed persons. He then examined their effects on plant growth.

Grad was attempting to demonstrate that there is an actual energetic effect that occurs in healing, which is unrelated to charisma or psychic ability. To do this, he used seedlings that were damaged in salt water and had healers hold the water that was later used on the plants. These plants grew stronger and more plentiful than the control seedlings. He further demonstrated that depressed patients produced negative effects on the growth of plants (Grad, 1979).

The Japanese researcher Motoyama developed a machine that electrically measured the acupuncture meridians for diagnosis in acupuncture treatment. Meridians are the energy flow lines coursing through the physical body that are studied and manipulated in acupuncture treatment. His 1981 study of energy, called *ki* in Japanese, found that meridians seem to exist in the dermal layer of connective tissue and have a direction of flow that can be detected. *Yin* energy flows upward; *yang* energy moves downward. The *ki* energy flows more slowly than galvanic skin response and nervous conduction. The *ki* also gathers in an affected meridian or organ, undergoes a transduction into a physiochemical energy or action potential, and can be detected by some individuals through sensory nerves. There seems to be a high center in the brain that controls the *ki* energy movement, according to Motoyama. The energy is also controlled by general physiochemical laws. When energy is flowing in different directions than it is supposed to, it is slowed down. Reverse flows have a lower amount of *ki* energy, whereas an excess of *ki* flows more rapidly (Motoyama, 1989, p. 257–268).

## Uses of Electricity in Healing

Another application of energetic concepts in medicine is the use of electricity to promote healing and to reduce pain. In the past two decades the orthopedist Robert Becker has measured direct current control systems in relation to the human body in health and disease. His most revolutionary work was stimulating the body's tissue to regenerate bone (Becker, 1990). He also stimulated regeneration of frog's limbs, which normally does not occur, by reversing the polarity of the electrical charge. Dr. Becker also demonstrated repair of compound fractures of horses by implanting bone electrodes in the cast, which pulsed currents across fracture sites. Other specialists (Stavish & Horwitz, 1987; Taubes, 1986) used electric currents to reduce tumor size and to clear cancers in difficult places to treat such as in the lung.

Therapy with the use of magnets has also been found helpful in rheumatoid and degenerative arthritis (Rose, 1987). Magnets were placed on either side of joints for one or two treatments per day for 10 to 15 sessions on nearly 200 rheumatoid and degenerative arthritic patients. Results showed improvement in 73% of the rheumatoid patients and in 67% of the degenerative joint patients.

Norman Shealey, MD, (1979) developed the Dorsal Column Stimulator, which utilized a weak electric current to alleviate intractable pain syndromes. This stimulator was surgically placed in the patient's lower spine to close the pain gate. Less intrusive pain gate closers have been developed since, such as the transcutaneous nerve stimulators that also use electricity to diminish pain sensation (Gerber, 2001).

# ENERGY UTILIZATION IN MEDICINE

There are many other forms of energy utilization in medicine. Madame Curie's discovery of radium led to the widespread use of X rays, which are also energetic phenomena (Gerber, 2001). CAT scans and MRI techniques track hydrogen atoms in the body, and images of their energetic emanations are interpreted by computers to yield a picture of the body's functioning. Zimmerman used the ultrasensitive SQUID (superconducting quantum interference device) to detect weak but significant increases in the magnetic field emanations of healers' hands during healing. He also measured brain waves, finding a right to left brain synchronization in the alpha, or meditative, state. He conjectures that grounding techniques, which healers use to focus themselves, are a connection into the earth's magnetic field to develop a synchronization of the healers' brain waves with the frequency of the earth's electromagnetic envelope (Brennan, 1993, p. 17).

Kirlian photography, a special photographic process that allows a direct image of the body's energy to be seen on sensitive film, (Moss, 1979) has been found to be useful in detecting cancer. Probes are placed over the body, and changes in frequency and polarity of the corona around the body allow disturbances to be detected (Gerber, 2001). It is quite possible that, in the near future, medical diagnosis of internal events may be done by assessing the etheric energy field.

## Brain Wave Patterns in Healers

Puharich measured a life-enhancing alternating magnetic field, at an 8-hertz rhythm, emanating from healers' hands. In his observations, increased or decreased frequencies seemed detrimental to life. Dr. Robert Beck, a nuclear physicist, found that the brain waves of healers across many groups and cultures exhibit the same brain-wave pattern, 7.8–8 hertz, when giving healing. These energy patterns fluctuate with the earth's magnetic field resonance of 7.8–8 hertz, which are called Schumann waves. Healers' brains synchronize both in frequency and phase with the Schumann waves; this is called field coupling. This coupling appears to provide access to a large field of energy for the work of healing (Brennan, 1993, p. 18).

A Polish healer, Mietek Wirkus, who has been a healer since childhood, has been monitored in a room isolated with copper walls. Dr. Elmer Green and Professor Fahrion of the Menninger Clinic, Topeka, KS, found increases of electrical surges, some of which registered eight volts or more, when Wirkus would initiate and send a charge of energy (Harpur, 1994).

Comparisons of energetic patterns in the biofield are being made across medical diagnoses through practitioners' reports of cases (Scandrett-Hibdon, Hardy, Mentgen, 2000). Protocols used by these practitioners are being studied to extract which intervention combinations seemed to affect the biofields the most.

# THE ENDOGENOUS HEALING PROCESS: A MODEL OF HEALING

Healing is mentioned in professional literature in limited ways, focusing primarily on the healer, healing techniques, and wound healing. Healing involves individuals in their own process. In other words, only clients can heal themselves. We haves observed six separate elements occurring in healing in which individuals move from disharmonious to harmonious patterns. These elements, which comprise the endogenous healing process, include:

1. Awareness
2. Appraisal
3. Choosing
4. Acceptance
5. Alignment
6. Outcome

Let's examine each of these aspects of the endogenous healing process (Scandrett-Hibdon & Freel, 1989) in more depth.

## Awareness

Awareness is the alerting mechanism that cues individuals to events within their internal and external environments. The disturbance may be physical, emotional, mental, or spiritual and is often perceived internally by the client. The cue is sometimes a vibrational one to disturbances in the energy field. Awareness is critical to any healing process because if we are not aware of an issue, it cannot be addressed for change.

As an example of awareness, we consider the case of a client who was being interviewed and reported being aware of fatigue, irritability, and pain. She was aware that something was amiss because, in her own words, "I feel like I'm dragging, many times I'm barking at the kids, and I know for sure that something isn't right."

## Appraisal

The second element in the endogenous healing process is appraisal. In appraisal, the individual explores and evaluates what awareness has brought to consciousness, assigns meaning to the disruption or cues, and makes comparisons with previous experiences, both from one's own knowledge and that of others. This knowledge may involve health information from a variety of sources.

To gain a greater understanding of appraisal, we look at the example of a physician who was also seeking help as a client. He knew something was wrong and tried to compare the symptoms with some of his previous experiences. He examined various syndromes of which he was aware and knew that this time his symptoms were different. He was using his expert knowledge to try to appraise the situation. After 3 to 4 weeks, when nothing shifted, he knew it was beyond the scope of his previous experiences and sought further medical and psychological help.

In other situations of appraisal, people know right away what the symptoms are and what to do. In these instances, they can go from awareness to appraisal and on to decision-making, basing the action on their appraisal.

# Choosing

From appraisal emerges a sense of clarity with which one can choose and set goals to handle the disharmony. In choosing, a client often makes decisions quickly without focusing much energy on them, as though from the subconscious. Thus, the decision can be inferred by observing the client's actions rather than by waiting for a cognitive statement. Some individuals choose to use the disharmony as an opportunity to learn, and they consciously involve themselves in examining all of the life pattern implications of the illness. Some clients choose to avoid focusing on the disharmony altogether; still others allow the disharmony to run its course or simply choose to yield to its disturbance.

# Acceptance

Acceptance might be considered to be a further aspect of choosing. In the process of "letting go," or deciding to accept, tension is released and relaxation occurs. With relaxation, energy shifts more easily so that repatterning to a more healthy state can occur with less effort.

In research, acceptance can be readily seen in catastrophically ill individuals. For example, one young woman reported having double pneumonia with concurrent bacterial and viral infections. As she lay in intensive care and was responding poorly to her medical regime, she reported reaching a point in her illness where she simply released herself to her Higher Power, explaining that she felt it did not matter whether she lived or died. With this release, she began to recover more quickly.

Acceptance, then, is associated with making choices and yielding to changes. Three main characteristics of acceptance seem to apply: (1) giving in to what is occurring, (2) letting go or ceasing to fix the disturbance, and (3) surrendering or passing responsibility of control to another, such as to a health care provider or Higher Power. Nonacceptance, on the other hand, occurs with a "fight it off" stance or with denial that any disturbance exists.

# Alignment

Alignment allows for the integration of the internal and external actions that support the movement toward harmony. In alignment, the energy shifts toward the goal of healing. Actions include activities such as changing one's diet, resting, or leaving uncomfortable situations. For example, a client stated, "To have ease in my life, I may need to leave a stressful job."

# Outcome

The endpoint or outcome of healing is a sense of being in harmony and experiencing a sense of wholeness. Healing, like health and illness, is value related and defined by clients in their own terms (Barrett, 1990). Informants reported that they clearly knew when they were healed. Descriptors that might be anticipated with healing include physical and psychological comfort, vitality, a sense of peace, and an inner knowing of wellness. These findings are part of research studies of endogenous healing (Scandrett-Hibdon, 1988, 1989, 1990).

***Model of the Endogenous Healing Process***    We can now look at a model of the endogenous healing process with the elements we have named in table 2.3.

| TABLE 2.3    **The Endogenous Healing Process** |
| --- |
| AWARENESS<br>    physical cues<br>    emotional cues<br>    mental and spiritual cues |
| APPRAISAL<br>    evaluating<br>    comparing with previous learning<br>    assigning meaning to the disruption |
| CHOOSING<br>    setting goal |
| ACCEPTANCE<br>    yielding, turning it over, or nonaccepting |
| ALIGNMENT<br>    internal and external actions |
| OUTCOME<br>    harmony<br>    experience of wholeness |

# ENDOGENOUS HEALING COMPARED WITH ESTABLISHED SYMPTOM RESPONSE PATTERNS

As we examine the literature on human responses to illness and disharmonious patterns, we see two major models. One may be described as a symptom response model based on sociological studies of illness behavior (Chrisman, 1977; Kasl & Cobb, 1966; Suchman, 1965; Zola, 1964) and is characterized by the simple seeking of symptom relief. The other is more psychologically oriented and involves learning better coping skills. This approach is often encompassed in coping or stress management strategies (Cohen & Lazarus, 1973; Lazarus & Folkman, 1984).

| TABLE 2.4 | Comparison of Healing, Coping, and Illness Response Models |||
|---|---|---|---|
| **ENDOGENOUS HEALING PROCESS** | **COPING MODEL** | **ILLNESS RESPONSE MODEL** ||
| Awareness<br>    physical<br>    emotional | – | presymptom cue<br>symptom recognition ||
| Appraisal<br>    evaluate<br>    compare<br>    assign meaning | cognitive appraisal<br>adequate response<br>    repertoire<br>judgment<br>discrimination<br>choice of activity | evaluation<br>labeling<br>monitoring ||
| Choosing<br>    denial<br>    fight it off<br>    treatment<br>    let go<br>    inferred from action | deployment of coping<br>    mechanisms | symptom definition<br>social environment<br>    for resources and<br>    treatment ||
| Acceptance | – | – ||
| Alignment<br>    self-action<br>    others' actions | recovery from stress | treatment of symptoms ||
| Outcome<br>    harmony<br>    well-being<br>    peace<br>    vitality | absence of stress | absence of symptoms ||

Neither of these more established models has been compared to the actual healing process, which we now understand to be more integrative and client centered. In table 2.4 we compare the endogenous healing process with the coping model and the illness response model to note the differences. As we can see, the coping and illness response models report observed behaviors without exploring the client's inner experience, commitment, or participation. In other words, acceptance and the possibility of aligning with resources and action are missing. The outcomes, therefore, are also quite different.

## SUMMARY

This brief history indicates a wide variety of human experiences with healing beyond mere symptom removal or coping with stress. The innate healing potential within the client needs to be honored by the facilitator, who can help and assist the endogenous process that we have described. The transformational view of healing suggests that the client gains a new perspective through awareness, appraisal, choosing, accepting, and aligning.

Energetic interventions that work with the human energy field allow the sensitivity and respect for the client's choices that can foster activation of the healing potential. The history of energy-oriented healing ranges from simple "laying on of hands" to working with the human energy field and more sophisticated measurements of the aura as we have discussed in this chapter.

We will explore biofield theory and its practical applications in Section II, but first we want to consider the most pertinent research related to energy-based healing. All of the history and research indicate we are yet at the very beginning of full understanding and investigation of this vitally important work.

## REFERENCES

Barrett, E. A. M. (1990). Health patterning with clients in a private practice environment. In M. Barrett (Ed.), *Visions of Rogers' science-based nursing*. New York: National League for Nursing.

Becker, R. (1990). *Cross Currents*. New York: Tarcher/Putnam.

Brennan, B. A. (1993). *Light emerging: The journey of personal healing*. New York: Bantam Books.

Bruyere, R., & Farrens, J. (1989). *Wheels of light: A study of the chakras*. San Madre, CA: Bon Publishers.

Chrisman, N. J. (1977). The health seeking process: An approach to the natural history of illness. *Culture Medicine Psychiatry, 1,* 351–377.

Cohen, F., & Lazarus, R. S. (1973). Active coping processes, coping dispositions, and recovery from surgery. *Psychosomatic Medicine, 35,* 375–389.

Elkin, A. P. C. (1978). *Aboriginal men of high degree.* New York: St. Martin's Press.

Gerber, R. (2001). *Vibrational medicine,* 3rd Ed., Rochester, VT: Bear & Co.

Grad, B. (1979). Some biological effects of laying on of hands and their implications. In Otto and Knights (Eds.), *Dimensions in wholistic healing: New frontiers in the treatment of the whole person.* Chicago: Nelson-Hall.

Guttenberg, E. (1997). *Daughter of the shaman.* New York, NY: Harper Prism.

Harpur, T. (1994). *The uncommon touch: An investigation of spiritual healing.* Toronto, Ontario: McClelland and Steward, Inc.

Hover-Kramer, D. (1993). *Energetic impressions of Egypt.* Poway, CA: Behavioral Health Consultants.

Kasl, S. V., & Cobb, S. (1966). Health behavior, illness behavior, and sick behavior: Part I. *Archives of Environmental Health, 13,* 246–266; Part II. Sick role behavior. *Archives of Environmental Health,* 13, 531–541.

Katz, R. (1982). *Boiling energy: Community healing among the Kalahari Kung.* Cambridge, MA: Harvard University Press.

Katz, R., Biesele, M. & St. Denis, V. (1997). *Healing makes our hearts happy.* Rochester, VT: Inner Traditions.

Keegan, L. (1988). The history and future of healing. In *Holistic nursing: A handbook for practice.* Rockville, MD: Aspen Publishers.

Kharitidi, L. (1996). *Entering the circle.* San Francisco, CA: Harper.

Krieger, D. (1987). *Living the Therapeutic Touch.* New York: Dodd, Mead and Company.

Landy, D. (1977). *Culture, disease and healing: Studies on medical anthropology.* New York: Macmillan.

Lazarus, R. S., & Folkman, S. (1984). *Stress, appraisal and coping.* New York: Springer Publishing Company.

Moss, T. (1979). *The body electric.* Los Angeles: J. P. Tarcher, Inc.

Motoyama, H. (1989). *Theories of the chakras.* Wheaton, IL: Theosophical Publishing House.

Ostrander, S., & Schroeder, L. (1977). *Psychic discoveries behind the iron curtain.* New York: Bantam.

Pavek, R. (1993). *Manual healing methods: Physical and biofield* (Report). Washington, DC; National Institute of Health — Office of Alternative Medicine.

Plotkin, M. J. (1993) *Tales of a shaman's apprentice.* New York, NY: Viking.

Quinn, J. F. (1992). Holding sacred space: The nurse as healing environment. *Holistic Nursing Practice, 6*(4), 26–36.

Rawnsley, M. M. (1985). Health: A Rogerian perspective. *Journal of Holistic Nursing, 3* (1), 13–26.

Rose, R. (1987, June 3). Magnetic pulses in RA: Less pain and mobility gain. *Medical Tribune.*

Rose, B. H. C., and Keegan, L. (2000). Exercise and movement. In Dossey, B. M., Keegan, L., and Buzetta, C. E. (Eds.), *Holistic nursing.* 3rd ed., Gaithersburg, MD: Aspen.

Rush, J. E. (1981). *Towards a general theory of healing.* Washington, DC: University Press of America.

Scandrett-Hibdon, S. (1988, February). *The endogenous healing process in elderly black women.* Study presented at second annual conference of the Southern Nursing Research Society, Atlanta, GA.

Scandrett-Hibdon, S. (1990). The endogenous healing process in adult women. *Journal of Holistic Nursing, 8*(1), 47–62.

Scandrett-Hibdon, S., & Freel, M. (1989). The endogenous healing process: Conceptual analysis. *Journal of Holistic Nursing, 7*(1), 66–72.

Scandrett-Hibdon, S., Hardy, C., and Mentgen, J. (2000). *Energetic patterns: Healing touch cases,* Vol I. Lakewood, CO: CO Center for Healing Touch.

Shealey, N. (1979). Wholistic healing and the relief of pain. In Otto and Knights (Eds.), *Dimensions of wholistic healing: New frontiers in the treatment of the whole person.* Chicago: Nelson-Hall.

Smith, L. L. (2000). *Called into healing.* Arvada, CO: Healing Touch Spiritual Ministries Press.

Stavish, S., & Horwitz, N. (1987, March 11). Pioneering cancer electrotherapy. *Medical Tribune.*

Suchman, E. A. (1965). Stages of illness and medical care. *Journal of Health and Human Behavior, 6,* 114–128.

Taubes, G. (1986). One electrifying possibility. *Discover.*

Veth, I. (1949). *The yellow emperor's classic of internal medicine.* Berkeley, CA: University of California Press.

Villodo, A. (2000). *Spirit medicine.* New York: Random House.

Zola, I. K. (1964). Illness behavior of the working class: Implications and recommendations. In A. Shostak, & W. Gomberg (Eds.), *Blue collar work: Studies of the American worker.* Englewood Cliffs, NJ: Prentice-Hall.

# CHAPTER 3

# Research Related
# to Healing Touch (HT)

*Norma Geddes, PhD, RN*

> *"Then one day you find someone who listens, who loves, someone gentle who feels your presence, and you start gradually to exist again, to feel, to trust, to be a genuine person."*
>
> —Moustakas, 1977, p. 94.

## INTRODUCTION

In the first edition of this book none of the research studies relating to energy-based healing used Healing Touch modalities as the independent variable. The research in Therapeutic Touch was the existing basis for the practice of energy-oriented modalities. These Therapeutic Touch studies helped us to understand some of the applications of energy healing in such areas as relieving pain and anxiety (Heidt, 1981, 1991; Quinn, 1984, 1989; Randolph, 1984; Keller & Bzdek, 1986; Meehan, 1993; Simington & Laing,1993; Gagne & Toye, 1994; Olson & Sneed, 1995; Peck, 1997; Turner et al., 1998), enhancing immune function (Quinn & Strelkauskas, 1993), and accelerating wound healing (Wirth, 1990).

Much has changed in the past five years. For one, there has been a conspicuous paradigm shift in research methodology, at least in the social sciences and nursing, as evidenced in the collection of *qualitative* as well as *quantitative* data about human experience. Each of these research approaches is set in a paradigm, a context, that holds assumptions about the interactive world and provides both theoretical and methodological direction (Creswell, 1994). Quantitative studies are an inquiry into a human problem based on testing a theory composed of variables, measured with numbers and analyzed with statistical procedures in order to determine whether the predictive generalizations of the theory hold true.

In contrast, qualitative studies are an inquiry into a human problem or situation based on building a complex picture and are conducted in natural settings to capture the informant's lived experience (Creswell, 1994). In other words, the collection of quantitative data consists of counting and measuring interventions that a researcher hypothesizes will or will not make a difference in a specified outcome. On the other hand, qualitative data is collected in order to find the meaning of certain human experiences. This data exists in all of the multiple ways that human beings express meaning, such as conversation, visual expression, music, art, poetry, journaling, and reflective dialogue. These data are collected through interviews, biographies, observation, a review of mementos, video/film footage, etc. There are various ways of organizing qualitative data in Healing Touch research, but the end result is a product that captures the essence of the HT experience. Both practitioners and researchers of HT agree that HT is a therapeutic encounter focused on facilitating healing in the direction of the recipient's highest good.

## LIMITATIONS OF QUANTITATIVE DATA

Quantitative data in HT research, like the more quantitative studies of TT named above, seek to show efficacy in relation to a decrease of such troublesome symptoms as pain and anxiety. The "gold standard" of a randomized, controlled trial of quantitative scientific inquiry is woefully insufficient in capturing the healing experience from either the recipient's or the practitioner's perspective. In quantitative studies, there is considerable planning to try to exclude any other variable than the main intervention as a cause of the treatment effect. Thus, the presence of practitioner consciousness, intent, centering, and other subtle qualities of the healing interaction are by definition excluded in quantitative research.

In HT research it is not possible to say that HT is the total explanation for facilitating relaxation or decreasing pain. In fact, the relaxation that usually follows HT sessions may be attributable to the caring presence of the practitioner, a change in breathing pattern, a change in awareness about a personal situation, or other causes. The phrase that quantitative researchers use for ruling out other explanations as the cause for a treatment result is "controlling for extraneous variables." Critics of energy-based healing deem the lack of control for extraneous variables a major research flaw. They also criticize poorly defined research terms, small sample sizes, and results from some studies that do not show "statistical significance" (meaning that the results of the study could just as easily have occurred by chance as by the healing method used). The Healing Touch response to these critics is not just to "clean up" or develop more quantitative studies, but to embrace the possibility of understanding the healing experience in ways that transcend counting and statistical analysis. This approach is necessary because conducting quantitative HT research is in dissonance with its theoretical frameworks, such as the Rogerian orientation to man as an indivisible energetic being co-existent with the universe. The quantitative findings satisfy the critics of energy-based healing modalities who say, "Ha! We knew there was nothing to this stuff!" But, more importantly, research framed in the quantitative paradigm simply misses the essence of the healing interaction.

There is a tendency to value research studies that support what we intuitively know to be true and to dismiss studies that are contrary to our own experience. Both these tendencies create problems in that we miss the chance to be influenced along new lines of thinking and we risk becoming complacent by failing to question our beliefs. A compromise to the problems inherent in the measurement of HT efficacy might be to include qualitative data in any study that is also trying to quantify results of an HT regimen. The consistent imperative remains that research to describe or measure HT cannot have a prescribed time frame or a prescribed regimen if one really wants to be faithful to the full possibilities of a healing encounter.

At the heart of the HT encounter is the experience of relationship between the practitioner and the recipient. The practitioner uses both specific techniques and intuitive awareness to facilitate healing. What we are learning through HT research is that this healing encounter has describable outcomes that are positive, nurturing, and desirable. I recall asking a woman whom I had been seeing on a weekly basis for almost a year, to help me understand how she experienced the HT part of our interaction. I wondered, for instance, if it were the caring presence, or my undivided attention that was actually the basis for her continuing to meet with me. She very quietly said, "There is something very important that happens with the energy part of it, but I can't explain it in words. The sensations are pre-verbal for me." Such outcomes do not lend themselves easily to quantifiable data.

## HEALING TOUCH INTERNATIONAL, INC. (HTI)

Healing Touch International, Inc. (HTI) has a designated research director and the office produces an annual survey which describes research in various stages of implementation and evaluation. In addition, this office provides information on sources of research funding support and networking information to practitioners with specific research interests. A listing of current HT research topics and contact people is provided in table 3.1.

In this chapter, we will present examples of HT research from the Healing Touch International (HTI) Year 2000 Survey. Four research studies will be described in detail and serve as exemplars of studies that address issues of efficacy as well as practitioner experience. There are numerous implications of HT research, and some of these will be discussed in relation to novice practitioners, experienced practitioners, health care workers in general, the HT program, and the need for future research.

| TABLE 3.1 | Listing of Healing Touch International Research Topics, 2000 |
| --- | --- |

(See Appendix B for contact Information)

| NAME | DATE | TITLE |
| --- | --- | --- |
| Brannon, Judy | 1997 | A patient satisfaction survey for cancer patients experiencing Healing Touch at the Cancer Wellness Center |
| Chapman, Catherine | 1998 | Energy-based psychotherapy in the context of the theories of Caroline Myss |
| Christiano, Charlene | 1997 | The lived experience of HT with cancer patients |
| Cordes, Pamela & Proffitt, Charlotte | 1998 | The effect of Healing Touch on the pain and joint mobility experienced by patients with total knee replacements |
| Darbonne, Madelyn & Fontenot, Tamara | 1997 | The effect of HT modalities on patients with chronic pain |
| Dubrey, Sr. Rita Jean | 1997 | A quality assurance project on the effectiveness of Healing Touch treatments as perceived by patients at the Wellness Institute |
| Forsman, Sandy | 1999 | The Healing Touch experience in elderly home care clients |
| Geddes, Norma | 1999 | The experience of personal transformation in Healing Touch practitioners |
| Leb, Cathy | 1997 | The effects of Healing Touch on depression |
| McAdams, Kathleen | 1998 | The effects of Healing Touch on cardiovascular and oxygenation variables in critically ill patients |
| Merritt, Patricia | 2000 | The effect of Healing Touch and other complementary therapies on diabetes |
| Merritt, Patricia & Randall, David | 2000 | Pilot program to study the effects of Healing Touch and other forms of energy work on cancer pain |
| Moreland, Kathy | 1997 | The lived experience of receiving the Chakra Connection of women with breast cancer who are receiving chemotherapy |
| Osterlund, Hob | 2000 | The "HeToBa" Study: Healing Touch for backs |
| Philpy, Sylvia & Hutchison, Cynthia | 1997 | The HEALTH Tool (Healing Energy and Life through Holism) |

(continues)

| TABLE 3.1 | Listing of Healing Touch International Research Topics, 2000 (continued) |

(See Appendix B for contact Information)

| NAME | DATE | TITLE |
|---|---|---|
| Robbins, Jo Lynne | 1999 | Psychoneuroimmunology and Healing Touch in HIV disease |
| Scheel, Nancy | 2000 | The development and initial testing of an instrument to assess advanced practice nursing graduate students' attitudes toward Healing Touch |
| Silva, M.A.C | 1996 | The effect of relaxation (HT) touch on the recovery level of postanesthesia abdominal hysterectomy patients. Reported in *Alternative Therapies, 96* (2), No. 4. |
| Slater, Vicki | 1995 | Safety, elements, and effects of Healing Touch on chronic non-malignant abdominal pain |
| Stouffer, D.,C., Kaiser, D., Pitman, G. & Rolf, W. | 2000 | Electrodermal testing to measure the effect of a Healing Touch treatment |
| Verret, Peggy | 1999 | Healing Touch as a relaxation intervention in children with spasticity |
| Wang, Kris, & Herman, Carol | 1999 | Healing Touch on agitation levels related to Dementia |
| Wardell, Diane | 1998 | Spirituality in Healing Touch practitioners: A comparison of spirituality between the participants in all the levels of the Healing Touch program |
| Wardell, Diane | 2000 | Trauma release technique as taught and experienced in the Healing Touch program. Published in *2000 Complementary and Alternative Therapies.* 6-1, 17-20. |
| Wetzel, Wendy | 1993 | Healing Touch as a nursing intervention: Wound infection following cesarean birth – An anecdotal case study. *Journal of Holistic Nursing, 11* (3). |
| Wheeler, Jo Lynne | 1996 | Data collection on the use of HT modalities with HIV+ patients |
| Wilkinson, Dawn, et. al. | 2000 | The effect of HT on salivary immunoglobulin A: Toward an understanding of energetic healing |

# OVERVIEW OF HT RESEARCH TOPICS

The January 2000 HTI Research Survey describes 27 research projects that have been completed or are in the process of data collection. The study topics include: a) issues of patient satisfaction, b) efficacy in a variety of clinical situations, c) miscellaneous topics. To summarize, the two research activities in Table 3.1 focus on patient satisfaction surveys by Brannon and Osterlund. Efficacy studies include: HT and patients with cancer by Christiano, Merritt, and Moreland; the effect of HT on pain and joint mobility in patients who have had total knee replacements by Cordes & Proffitt; HT and chronic pain by Darbonne & Fontenot, and Slater; HT and post-operative recovery by Silva; HT and the elderly by Forsman; HT and depression by Leb; HT and the effect on cardiovascular and oxygenation variables in critically ill patients by McAdams; HT and diabetes by Merritt; HT and children with spasticity by Verret; HT and dementia by Wang & Hermann; trauma release as taught and experienced in the HT program by Wardell; HT and clients with HIV by Wheeler and Robbins.

Several activities have included the development of research tools for data collection: a documentation tool for use during HT sessions by Philpy & Hutchison; and a documentation tool for client assessment of attitudes related to HT by Scheel.

Research studies that focus on the practitioner include the experience of personal transformation by Geddes and a comparison of spirituality between participants in all levels of the HT program by Wardell.

Miscellaneous topics include: theoretical linkages between energy-based psychotherapy and the work of Caroline Myss by Chapman; electrodermal testing to measure the effect of HT by Stouffer, et al.; HT as a quality assurance initiative at a wellness institute by Dubrey.

## Examples of Healing Touch Research

Four research studies will now be described in more detail and will serve as exemplars of current Healing Touch research activity.

***The Effectiveness of Healing Touch in Enhancing Health***    Conducted by Wilkinson, Knox, Chatman, Johnson, Barbour, Miles, and Reel in 1999, this study incorporates both qualitative and quantitative data with a sample size of 22. The multidisciplinary research team from Tennessee State University included a doctoral student in counseling psychology, faculty in the department of psychology, a biologist, a biology laboratory supervisor, and nurses. Unlike studies that use a prescribed regimen of HT, and a prescribed time frame, this study allowed for the "normal and customary practice" of the discipline.

The research objectives were: a) to determine whether HT enhances health in clients in terms of immunocompetence, self-reporting of stress levels, and perceptions of health enhancement and the HT experience; and, b) to determine whether training and experience level of the practitioner is relevant to treatment efficacy. The participants in this study were 22 clients who had never had HT and 9 practitioners of varying training levels. Four of the nine practitioners were either certified or had completed IIIA level of training. Three practitioners had completed IIB, one had completed IIA, and one had completed training at level I. The three treatment conditions were: no treatment, HT only, and HT with music and guided imagery. Outcome measures were radial immunodiffusion of IgA concentrations in the saliva, questionnaires, and the HEALTH tool (Philpy & Hutchison, 1997). The results of this study show the following outcomes:

1. Clients whose practitioners had higher levels of training had significantly higher IgA after the "HT Only" condition as compared to the "No Treatment" condition, while clients whose practitioners had lower levels of training did not have significantly different IgA after HT treatment.

2. Clients reported a significant reduction of stress levels after both HT-linked conditions, regardless of the training level of their practitioners, while stress levels did not change in the "No Treatment" group.

3. Perceived enhancement of health was reported by 13 of the 22 clients (59.1%).

4. Themes of relaxation, connection, and enhanced awareness (including pain relief) were identified in questionnaire transcripts.

5. Fifteen of twenty-two participants (68.2%) responded positively on criteria that considered the effects of HT on a wide range of health concerns.

6. Beliefs and expectations about HT, as measured by placebo predictor questions, were unrelated to positive responses to treatment for this sample.

The researchers in this study concluded that the data support the use of HT by highly trained HT practitioners for health enhancement. They also concluded that the study needs to be replicated with a larger sample.

***Psychoneuroimmunology and Healing Touch in HIV Disease***    In 1999, Jo Lynne Robbins successfully defended her doctoral dissertation research, which was to ascertain the effects of HT on well-being and neuroendocrine function in individuals living with HIV disease. A total of 27 males completed four HT sessions, given on a weekly basis, which lasted for 30 minutes and consisted of only the Chakra Connection (process described in chapter 9). Because of the small sample size and the impact of gender on neuroendocrine and immune function, women were not included in the study. Dependent variables included well-being as measured by three well-being and two psychological distress instruments, serum serotonin, salivary DHEA and cortisol, and a variety of enumerative and functional measures of immune function. A pretest–posttest experimental design, including a wait-list control group, was used. The data were analyzed using conventional statistical methods for multiple variables. It was hypothesized that HT would increase participant well-being, serum serotonin, and salivary DHEA; decrease salivary cortisol; and improve immune function in individuals living with HIV disease. All of the research hypotheses were rejected.

This study is important because it exemplifies the predisposition of current researchers to follow the quantitative experimental method. At the same time, this study contains the design flaws that have been reported by researchers of quantitative Therapeutic Touch studies: small sample size, prescribed duration and regimen of intervention, and multiple confounding variables. Robbins reports in her dissertation that there were serendipitous results to the HT intervention that were not captured in her report on the formalized hypotheses. For instance, the majority of the HT recipients asked to continue HT treatment after the study concluded, and a free clinic has been established to meet that need. It appears, then, that the recipients experienced something that they considered worthwhile even though the quantitative data did not support the study hypotheses.

### The Experience of Personal Transformation in Healing Touch Pracititioners

In 1999, Norma Geddes, author of this chapter, completed her doctoral dissertation with the above named title.The study was a heuristic inquiry with eight certified Healing Touch practitioners. Data were collected by taped, transcribed interviews and through the researcher's observation in the HT program as a participant. The practitioners were considered co-researchers in the heuristic research process, which incorporated personal knowing of the researcher as a rich and relevant source of data. All of the data from the participants were analyzed and organized into themes, processes, individual depictions, a composite depiction, and a creative synthesis of the experience of personal transformation.

The experience of personal transformation in Healing Touch practitioners was described as a journey, not a destination. It was described as a process of making changes in all facets of life based on a perception of the self as a unitary, spiritual, self-caring, and self-nurturing being. The participants in the process of personal transformation were increasingly less dependent on the approval of others and strived to allow the people in their path the space they needed for their own growth. There were periods of solitude and introspection; periods of lively engagement with kindred souls; and periods of excitement and wonder at the deep capacity for feeling connected with an inner being, others, and a higher being.

Although each individual's story of personal transformation was unique, themes and processes emerged that were common to all. Three common themes were: (1) a perceived sense of "rightness" of the experience of Healing Touch despite diverse ways of being introduced to the program; (2) unanticipated personal implications; and (3) a new lens through which to view one's life and circumstances. Processes that added specificity to the first theme included: (a) a willingness to be open to a new experience, and (b) a recognition of the experience as exhilarating, curious, interesting, and compelling. Processes that added specificity to the second theme included changes in: (a) relationships, (b) employment, (c) housing, and (d) values—from a material to a spiritual focus. Processes that added specificity to the third theme included: (a) the experience of feelings, thoughts, and behaviors related to connection with a unitary being, others, and a higher being; (b) a new capacity for self-caring; (c) a new capacity to care for others in a non-judgmental way; (d) a contented stillness that is immediately available; and (e) a new appreciation for life as a source of curiosity, excitement, and mystery.

As well as descriptive data, the study contributed data for the relevance of the unitary paradigm and Newman's theory of health as expanding consciousness (Newman, 1994). This gives a theoretical orientation for understanding both the experience of personal transformation in HT practitioners, and the personal relationship that develops between the practitioner and the recipient in HT interactions.

Qualitative data describe possible human experiences and are intended at best to be applicable, not generalizable, to others. The data in this study describe both the commonalities and the unique experiences of personal transformation that were present for the researcher and for the eight HT practitioners. All of the practitioners were quite clear about the substantive, albeit not exclusive, relationship between the experience of being an HT practitioner and their personal transformation. As one participant described her journey:

> I think we're all from the same energy source and we're down here going to school, learning how to love each other. We're all in the same play together so to speak. We're tremendously interconnected. What I do to you, I'm really doing to myself. There's a whole set of universal laws, one of them being, what goes around, comes around. Not in the way that many people on the earth think of it but more in spiritual energetic terms. What goes out comes back … because of this tremendous interconnectedness that we have with each other and not only with each other but with the planet and everything on the planet too. All my beliefs about karma are weaved into that. I think it is all about evolution and it's all about developing, and if we aren't developing, if we're not doing what we need to do in this school of learning about love, the Universe will provide us with some very interesting opportunities to learn what is on our agenda. In fact, I believe that the Universe goes, "Yoo hoo, pay attention, you created this thing to learn and it's time now." If you say, "Thank you, but you know I'm going golfing or I'm busy making a million dollars or whatever," then the Universe will say harder, "Pay attention now. You're part of this." It's not like the Universe is doing this to you; you're part of this

process with your higher self. We have to evolve, otherwise we get into stuck energy and stuck energy is disease, being out of ease, and we get into all sorts of trouble unless we are evolving. It's about evolution.

*The "HeToBa" Study: Healing Touch for Backs*    A two year hospital study, called "Project Back" currently in progress at Queen's Medical Center in Hawaii, involves offering HT to employees with acute back injuries. It is headed by Hob Osterlund. This project was initiated following pilot work that indicated employee satisfaction and the potential for a positive financial savings for the hospital. The study design calls for 45 consenting employees with acute back injuries who would be randomized into 3 groups. One group would receive the Federal Agency for Health Care Policy and Research (AHCPR) guidelines approach only; the second group would receive HT within 72 hours of injury and two additional treatments; the third group would receive three relaxation sessions of the same duration as an HT treatment. Outcome measures for all three groups would evaluate the impact on medical costs, lost work time, pain levels, and functional abilities. In reviewing the findings of this study it will be important to know how confounding variables are controlled, and whether there is a significant difference in the outcome variables among the three groups. Data collection for this project began in January, 1999.

As of March, 2000, approximately 17 people had been enrolled in the study. Why such a low number after more than a year of initiating the research? There are two main reasons: staff members do not always report back injuries in a timely manner and the study protocol requires an early intervention soon after injury. The second reason is that HT is such a well-known healing modality at Queen's Medical Center that employees who are injured are not willing to let themselves be randomized into a group that does not receive HT care (Osterlund, personal communication, 4/28/00). The latter reason supports the need to explore the subjective meaning of the HT experience through qualitative studies that ask about inner satisfaction, in addition to efficacy issues, in evaluating the experience of HT.

# IMPLICATIONS OF HT RESEARCH

The implications and outcomes of HT research concern novice practitioners, experienced practitioners, health care workers, and the need for ongoing research. Some of these issues are discussed briefly.

## Novice and Experienced Practitioners

The HT program incorporates content related to caring for the self, and the potential for metaphysical experiences related to energy work (e.g., meditative states of consciousness; perceptions of energy fields which consist of being able to visualize light around a physical body). However, nothing quite prepares practitioners for the considerable positive changes that occur in the lives of new practitioners. For instance, this author notes (1999) that every one of the practitioners in her study wondered at some point if they were "nuts," "whacko," or having delusions! As one participant said, "I am a psychotherapist and I put people in the hospital for seeing things." The data in this and other studies therefore serve as an impetus for curriculum expansion related to the potential for personal transformation for participants in the HT program.

A tendency exists among caregivers to overextend themselves and lose sight of the many ways in which small acts of compassionate caring make a difference. An initial enthusiasm for healing processes may progress to a state of "burnout" if nurses and healers do not celebrate their "healing moments" (Dossey, Keegan, & Guzzetta, 2000). We have much to learn about easing caregiver burdens. Energy-based healing viewed from a unitary perspective serves both client and practitioner as a path to healing. Starn (1989) describes her initial impetus for becoming what she calls an "energy healer." She prayed, "God, I will go anywhere and do anything you ask me to do, if I can just heal this exhaustion and fatigue" (p. 209). Starn's later description of a healing encounter differs markedly from her "exhausted, fatigued" description of her earlier state: "In the relaxed, balanced state, energy healers become fully present, connect to the Universal Energy Field . . . and allow or channel the specific vibrations needed to help the client maintain or regain health, cope with chronic disease, or achieve a peaceful death" (p. 213).

Thus, the energy healer is relaxed, receptive to, and a conduit for Universal Energy. Practitioners are responsive to whatever serves the client's highest good. This view of the practitioner in a healing encounter is congruent with Rogers's unitary paradigm (Rogers, 1994a), Newman's theory of health as expanding consciousness (1994), and the American Nurses' Association Social Policy Statement. This document describes the following four values and assumptions:

"1. Humans manifest an essential unity of mind/body/spirit.
2. Human experience is contextually and culturally defined.
3. Health and illness are human experiences.
4. The presence of illness does not preclude health nor does optimal health preclude illness" (ANA, 1995, p. 3).

Experienced practitioners attest to the need for daily renewal of their sources of inspiration and comfort. Sources of comfort are unique to each individual, but both personal and work environments need to be conducive to the renewal process. As one HT practitioner has said about her personal environment, "There is no rationing of weird out here. I can do what I need to nourish my spirit." Data from research that focus on the practitioner serve to remind and inspire experienced practitioners to honor and care for themselves.

# Health Care Workers

Research and practice implications have arisen from the increased use of alternative therapies in the United States (Eisenberg et al., 1998). Selected data from telephone surveys conducted in 1997 are as follows:

1  The use of at least one of 16 alternative therapies increased from 33.3% in 1990 to 42.1% in 1997.

2. The therapies that increased the most were herbal medicine, massage, megavitamins, self-help groups, folk remedies, energy healing, and homeopathy.

3. There were no significant changes in disclosure (letting the primary care physician know of the use of alternative modalities), which was 39.8% in 1990 and 38.5% in 1997.

4. The total visits to alternative practitioners between 1990 and 1997 increased by 47.3% and exceeded visits to all U.S. primary care physicians.

There is considerable literature that describes the clinical use of alternative medicine. Some examples include clients with HIV infection (Evans, 1999), and patients with burns (Turner, et. al., 1998). As research in this area addresses other clinical applications, health care workers need to become informed about alternative and complementary care modalities. However, information alone is not sufficient. Changes in practice are needed: "Many natural, alternative, and complementary therapies offer relief, transcendence, and ease for many discomforts, and thus need to be part of our conventional treatment" (Huebscher, 1998b, p. 119). One implication for practice is that the experience of becoming involved in at least one form of alternative therapy, such as HT, has the potential to be personally rewarding and transformative to the caregiver.

As health care workers become more informed about alternative modalities and begin to incorporate them into their practice they will risk involvement in issues raised by the scientific community. For example, one issue is the need for testing: "What most sets alternative medicine apart . . . is that it has not been scientifically tested and its advocates largely deny the need for such testing" (Angell & Kassirer, 1998, p. 839). It is important for nurses to be clear about their involvement in alternative therapies that are part of their nursing practice domain, and to be able to distinguish valid nursing practice from exploratory alternative modalities. For instance, as we have seen over the last 10 years, HT is a modality that promotes relaxation, eases pain, and does no harm. Although research concerning its efficacy is ongoing, there may be many lost opportunities to ease suffering if the requirement for use is more rigorous quantitative scientific testing. As energy workers develop a specific knowledge base for healing modalities, it is for us to guide the decisions about which research questions to ask, which methods to use, and to determine what counts as evidence for research based practice.

# NEED FOR ONGOING RESEARCH

All of the completed and ongoing research projects related to HT stimulate further inquiry. Some interesting research questions emerge when looking at issues related to both practitioners and clients.

For instance, what role does cultural diversity, religious diversity, gender diversity, socioeconomic diversity, or age contribute to the experience of personal transformation in HT practitioners?  Is the experience of personal transformation in HT practitioners the same or different from the personal transformation experienced by practitioners of other complementary modalities? What happens over time in the experience of HT practitioners? Are the experiences of "rightness" with the healing role, of making lifestyle changes, and of viewing the world through a unitary lens sustained over time? Do HT practitioners sustain the view of themselves as unitary beings in whom spirituality is integral to their life experience? It would be interesting to interview the same practitioners in replicated studies at three to five years and ask them how their lives have changed. Any potential human experience that appears to enrich and enliven us, that nourishes our affinity with our inner being and with others, is worth learning about in great detail and is central to the healer's intention of serving the highest good of all.

In our Western society we have learned that technology is necessary but insufficient for survival. We also need human caring in all of its manifestations. Ongoing research is needed to evaluate clients' perceived experience related to pain and anxiety in light of both statistically significant and insignificant findings. We must continue to ask, what are the possible ways to account for the confounding variables on the efficacy of HT? In addition, client outcomes related to sense of well-being and increased immune function require ongoing study.

Evaluation of the theoretical bases for energy healing are another rich area for exploration. There is a need for ongoing theory and knowledge development concerning the following areas: (a) human energy fields, (b) Rogers's theory of unitary beings, (c) Newman's theory of health as expanding consciousness, and (d) questions about the HT recipients' experience that are not supported by statistical significance.

Reeder (1999) proposed the idea that a human energy field is a metaphor as opposed to an actual description of physical reality. She argues that research and education can advance by the use of this metaphor "to represent the revolutionary, fully pandimensional human being rather than as a literal entity connoting Newtonian three-dimensionality" (p. 7). The arena of quantum physics and the interconnectedness of all beings is no longer just discussed in the hallowed realm of academic physicists. Relevant books, TV programs, movies, and multi-media presentations are now very much in the public eye, with a plethora of references to angels, extraterrestial life, after-death experiences, and chaos theory.

While there is ongoing debate and study of human energy fields as real or metaphorical, the assumption of an "irreducible wholeness of humans as energy fields" (Rogers, 1994) is at the heart of energy-based healing research. One clinical application of Rogers's science of unitary human beings is unitary pattern appreciation "guided by participatory mutual engagement" (Cowling, 1999, p. 135). Participatory mutual engagement intended to facilitate unitary well-being is described by Barrett (1998) as "knowing participation in change" (p. 136). Cowling (1998) added specificity to the process of mutual engagement in knowing participation: "We come to knowing and appreciating pattern, our own and others' through focused engagement and with one another. . . . The instrument development in unitary case inquiry is the development of the researcher/practitioner's sensitivity to wholeness . . . throwing open the doors of human life and experience and knowing more fully than we ever imagined" (p.144). Martha Rogers specifically cited TT as one regimen that could facilitate health patterning in clients and personally experienced HT at the 1991 American Holistic Nurses' Association conference. The many healing modalities used by HT practitioners are instrumental in increasing the practitioners' sensitivity to wholeness. More studies are needed which detail the relationships among healing regimens, the practitioner/client dyad involved in knowing participation in change, and manifestations of unitary being and interconnection.

Recent nursing research studies that are theoretically based in Newman's work contain practical suggestions that could enhance future studies of HT practitioners. Several theorists (Yamashita,1998, 1999; and Yamashita & Tall, 1998) describe the need for follow-up interviews (perhaps one year after the original data collection) of individuals experiencing expanding consciousness in a healing intervention. This follow-up is needed to appreciate ongoing insight clients may have about their own "pattern, concomitant illumination, and possibilities for action" (Yamashita & Tall, 1998, p. 94). Geddes's (1999) study described the potential for the HT practitioner to make life changes in thought, behavior, feelings, relationships, employment, and living arrangements, which all contributed to an experience of expanding consciousness. A follow-up study in one year, or perhaps five years, of these same practitioners would help further explore this theoretical link.

## Combining Qualitative and Quantitative Data

A recent publication of a meta-analytic review of the effectiveness of TT revealed problems related to sampling procedures, intervention practices, practitioner skill, and underreporting of data (Peters, 1999, p. 58). The relevant finding from this meta-analysis is that practitioner data, including level of expertise and a description of the mutual process occurring between the client and practitioner, is useful information for assessing treatment outcomes. Therefore, there is a recommendation from multiple sources that quantitative studies include qualitative data of the practitioners' experience (Quinn & Strelkauskas, 1993; Meehan, 1993). Ongoing studies are needed that focus on many aspects of the practitioner's experience personally and in therapeutic encounters.

In contrast to the research described in this book's first edition, recent studies describe Therapeutic Touch as a potential "beneficial adjuvant nursing intervention" (Meehan, 1998). Pending further inquiry, "TT may become an important part of nursing care for hospitalized burn patients, as well as for other patients for whom pain and anxiety are major problems" (Turner, et. al., 1998, p. 20).

## SUMMARY

There is much to learn about the possibilities inherent in healing relationships. The burgeoning interest in alternative therapies and the increase in the numbers of HT practitioners in the past five years underscore the interest of consumers and the satisfaction of the practitioner. We must become our own staunchest advocates and our own sternest critics if we are to transcend the limiting quantitative paradigm and foster new ways of knowledge development. We may well develop ways of controlling for confounding variables in studies related to efficacy. Research that is grounded in randomized, controlled trials may be an effective HT future research methodology. To date this is not the case. This does not mean that we should just stare in wonder at the subjective expressions of pain relief and relaxation that recipients of HT often express. We do need to capture the essence of the HT experience in as many ways as humans express meaning in their lives. We need to support novice practitioners in their emergent awareness of a unitary world and we need to treasure the seasoned practitioners who need help in cultivating a sense of proportion in their giving and receiving. Research is about learning and unlearning, about building on new foundations, and about changing thoughts, feelings, and attitudes in light of new evidence and in light of new experience.

## REFERENCES

American Nurses'Association (ANA). (1995). *Nursing's social policy statement.* American Nurses Publishing: Washington, DC.

Angell, M. & Kassirer, J. P. (1998). Alternative medicine—The risks of untested and unregulated remedies. *The New England Journal of Medicine, 339* (12), 839–841.

Barrett, E. A. M. (1998). A Rogerian practice methodology for health patterning. *Nursing Science Quarterly, 11* (4), 136–138.

Cowling, W. R. (1998). Unitary case inquiry. *Nursing Science Quarterly, 11* (4), 139–141.

Cowling, W. R. (1999). A unitary-transformative nursing science: Potentials for transcending dichotomies. *Nursing Science Quarterly, 12* (2), 132–137.

Creswell, J. W. (1994). *Research design: Qualitative and quantitative approaches.* Thousand Oaks, CA: Sage.

Dossey, B. M., Keegan, L., & Guzzetta, C. E. (2000). *Holistic nursing: A handbook for practice.* (3rd ed.). Gaithersburg, MD: Aspen.

Eisenberg, D. M., Davis, R. B., Ettner, S. L., Appel, S., Wilkey, S., Van Rompay, M., & Kessler, R. (1998). Trends in alternative medicine use in the United States, 1990—1997: Results of a follow-up national survey. *The Journal of the American Medical Association, 280* (18), 1569–1575.

Evans, B. M. (1999). Complementary therapies and HIV infection. *American Journal of Nursing, 99* (2), 42–45.

Gagne, D., & Toye, R. C. (1994). The effects of therapeutic touch and relaxation therapy in reducing anxiety. *Archives of Psychiatric Nursing, VIII* (3), 184–189.

Heidt, P. R. (1981). Effect of therapeutic touch on the anxiety level of hospitalized patients. *Nursing Research, 30* (1), 32–37.

Heidt, P. R. (1991). Helping patients to rest: Clinical studies in therapeutic touch. *Holistic Nursing Practice, 5* (4), 57–66.

Hover-Kramer, D., Mentgen, J., & Scandrett-Hibdon, S. (1996) *Healing touch: A resource for health care professionals.* New York: Delmar.

Huebscher, R. (1998a). Alternative approaches. *Nurse Practitioner Forum, 9* (1) 1–2.

Huebscher, R. (1998b). Quality in natural/alternative/complementary health care practice. *Nurse Practitioner Forum, 9* (3), 119–120.

Keller, E., & Bzdek, V. M. (1986). Effects of therapeutic touch on tension headache pain. *Nursing Research, 35* (2), 101–106.

Meehan, T. C. (1993). Therapeutic touch and postoperative pain: A Rogerian research study. *Nursing Science Quarterly 6* (2), 69–78

Meehan, T. C. (1998). Therapeutic touch as a nursing intervention. *Journal of Advanced Nursing, 28* (1), 117–125.

Moustakas, C. E. (1977). *Creative life.* New York: Van Norstrand.

Moustakas, C. (1990). *Heuristic research: Design, methodology, and applications.* Newbury Park, CA: Sage.

Moustakas, C. (1994). *Phenomenological research methods.* Thousand Oaks: Sage.

Newman, M. A. (1986). *Health as expanding consciousness.* St. Louis: The C. V. Mosby Company.

Newman, M. A. (1994). *Health as expanding consciousness.* (2nd. ed.). New York: NLN Press.

Newman, M. A. (1997). Evolution of the theory of health as expanding consciousness. *Nursing Science Quarterly, 10* (1), 22–25.

Olson, M., & Sneed, N. (1995). Anxiety and therapeutic touch. *Issues in Mental Health Nursing, 16* (2), 97–108.

Peck, S. D. E. (1997). The effectiveness of therapeutic touch for decreasing pain in elders with degenerative arthritis. *Journal of Holistic Nursing, 15* (2), 176–198.

Peters, R. M. (1999). The effectiveness of therapeutic touch: A meta-analytic review. *Nursing Science Quarterly, 12* (1), 52–61.

Quinn, J. F. (1984). Therapeutic touch as energy exchange: Testing the theory. *Advances in Nursing Science, 6* (2), 42–49.

Quinn, J. F. (1989). Therapeutic touch as energy exchange: Replication and extension. *Nursing Science Quarterly, 2* (2), 79–87.

Quinn, J. F., & Strelkauskas, A. J. (1993). Psychoimmunologic effects of therapeutic touch on practitioners and recently bereaved recipients: A pilot study. *Advances in Nursing Science, 15* (4), 13–26.

Randolph, G. L. (1984). Therapeutic touch and physical touch: Physiological responses to stressful stimuli. *Nursing Research, 33* (1), 33–36.

Reeder, F. M. (1999). Energy: Its distinctive meanings. *Nursing Science Quarterly, 12* (1), 6–7.

Rogers, M. E. (1994a). The science of unitary human beings: Current perspectives. *Nursing Science Quarterly, 7* (1), 33–35.

Rogers, M. E. (1994b). Science of unitary being. In V. M. Malinski & E. A. M. Barrett (Eds.), *Martha E. Rogers: Her life and her work*. Philadelphia: F. A. Davis Co.

Simington, J. A., & Laing, G. P. (1993). Effects of therapeutic touch on anxiety in the institutionalized elderly. *Clinical Nursing Research, 2* (4), 438–450.

Starn, J. R. (1998). The path to becoming an energy healer. *Nurse Practitioner Forum, 9* (4), 209–216.

Steckel, C. M. & King, R. P. (1996). Therapeutic touch in the coronary care unit. *Cardiovascular Nursing, 10* (3), 50–54.

Turner, J. G., Clark, A. J., Gauthier, D. K., & Williams, M. (1998). The effect of therapeutic touch on pain and anxiety in burn patients. *Journal of Advanced Nursing, 28* (1), 10–20.

Wirth, D. T. (1990). The effect of non-contact therapeutic touch on the healing rate of full thickness dermal wounds. *Subtle Energies, 1* (1), 1–20.

Yamashita, M. (1998). Newman's theory of health as expanding consciousness: Research on family caregiving in mental illness in Japan. *Nursing Science Quarterly, 11* (3), 110–115.

Yamashita, M. (1999). Newman's theory of health applied in family caregiving in Canada. *Nursing Science Quarterly, 12* (1), 73-79.

Yamashita, M., Jensen, E., & Tall, F. (1998). Therapeutic touch: Applying Newman's theoretic approach. *Nursing Science Quarterly, 11* (2), 49–50.

Yamashita, M. & Tall, F. D. (1998). A commentary on Newman's theory of health as expanding consciousness. *Advances in Nursing Science, 21* (1), 65–75.

# The Human Energy System

*In this section we will explore the nature of the human energy system and its identified components—the biofield, the seven major energy centers, and the meridians. After exploring possible scientific bases for Healing Touch, we will describe the properties of the biofield and chakras and give implications of these concepts for assessment and intervention by the practitioner.*

# Toward an Understanding of the Scientific Bases of Healing Touch

*Victoria E. Slater, PhD, RN, CHTP/I, HNC*

> " ...We will never understand the scientific basis of everything. We must be open to approaches that work even when we don't understand how or why they work."
>
> —Ralph Snyderman, MD, Sept., 2000

## INTRODUCTION

Healing Touch (HT) practitioners know from their own experiences that HT can change lives. They have no question about it—HT assists bodies, minds, emotions, and spirits to heal. The question is how. From a Western scientific perspective, very little is known about how HT works, although research suggests a few avenues to explore. At this time, the mechanisms by which HT works must be inferred from people's experiences, which are often described in two ways. One set of descriptions sounds as if HT acts electrically; people use words like "frequency," "energy," and "vibration." The second set of descriptions is informational; both healer and client may experience images of the client's history, and after an HT treatment, clients will often understand or relate differently to their histories.

Physics suggests mechanics that may underpin HT, and HT providers know that the hand positions and motions used in the approach are not the whole picture. Practitioner centering and intention are key concepts, and consciousness research offers clues as to how they may influence HT results. This chapter will explore the mechanisms of HT from two perspectives: 1) the physical laws and structures suggested by the experience of the human biofield, chakras, and meridians, and 2) research on consciousness that may provide insight about how an HT provider may assist another's healing. Electrical and computer technology will be used as metaphors for human energy systems to make visible what is invisible to our five senses and to meet the empirical needs of Western minds.

# THE MECHANISMS OF HEALING TOUCH: WHAT IS SURMISED

It is important to keep in mind that nothing is known about how HT works. Human and non-human research results point to some avenues worth investigating, such as Zimmerman's (1990) studies of healers and meditators that suggest that HT's mechanism may be similar to pulsed electromagnetic fields (PEMF). How would a human produce such a field? That question is unanswered; some day the nature and effects of human electromagnetic fields, electrical currents, and magnetic fields will be common knowledge, but right now we must rely on reports of healers' and recipients' experiences to begin to understand the mechanisms of HT. Healers consistently describe HT using words like vibration, frequencies, resonance, and energy, as they discern information about the recipient's structural, physiological, emotional, mental, and spiritual problems. The mechanism of storage and retrieval of the information is unseen, somewhat like the hidden workings of a computer, which is an electromagnetic device.

The computer and other electromagnetic devices are useful metaphors to try to understand the mechanisms of HT. Because the mechanics of chakras and the aura, or biofield, are unknown, we are not able to say that the biofield "is" an electromagnetic field; we are only able to say that it "acts like" one. Similarly, chakras act like transformers, capacitors, and semiconductors. We know more about the mechanism underlying meridians, so we are able to say that they carry direct electric currents. We infer that they also carry information.

## A Primer on Electrical Devices

The best metaphors for human chakras, meridians, and biofields are electrical devices, which begin with moving electrons. A moving electron creates a wake of magnetic radiation, much like a speed boat puts out a wake in the water that frustrates novice water skiers and delights experts. Slow speed boats put out smaller wakes; faster ones put out stronger, taller, more powerful ones. The active component is the electron, and the resulting wake is called electromagnetic radiation, or light. Radiation is measured by the number of waves, or cycles per second (frequency); the height of the wave is called the amplitude. AM radio stations modify the amplitude of the wavelength of light to send music; FM stations change the frequency. When two speed boats pass each other, their wakes will collide, creating a larger wake. In the case of electrons, both the amplitude and frequency may change as they pass each other.

Electrical currents and magnetic fields affect each other—an electrical current creates a magnetic field and a magnetic field will influence an adjacent electrical current. If the electrical flow going through one wire is *changing*, its changing magnetic field will stimulate a current in an adjacent wire; the new current is called an induced current. Induced currents are an efficient way to create more power from a relatively tiny initial input. This simple process can be adapted in a variety of ways. It can be used to transform electricity so you can light and heat your home, talk on the telephone, and receive your favorite radio or television station.

Induced currents may be the mechanism behind many HT techniques. As HT practitioners sweep the recipient's body with their fingers, they are passing a pulsed electromagnetic field near the weak direct currents (DC) in the meridians. The effect, then, may be a more more powerful meridian flow, which enables the entire body to relax.

Electrical currents are not perpetual; they must be maintained. The unidirectional flow of electrons in a DC current slows down because of the friction of the electrons interacting with each other and with the walls of the wire. A DC current is like a traffic jam at 5:00 on the Friday before a holiday weekend. When everyone is going the same direction, the traffic comes to a standstill. DC currents need to be boosted or changed to stay alive. To avoid the slowing down of electrons, engineers developed an alternating current (AC). AC currents are always changing, and changing currents in one wire will induce a current in a second wire. A relatively small amount of changing electricity can induce more electricity and provide relatively inexpensive power. The current in your home reverses direction 120 times per second (Gonick & Huffman, 1990, p. 180). For currents to continue to flow, they either need to be boosted, as the acupoints boost the meridians, or changed, as in alternating electrical flow patterns of the chakras.

To increase the secondary current's strength still further, we can modify the magnetic field by winding the electrical wire into a coil (called a solenoid) that will look something like the loops on a telephone cord. We can alter the solenoid's strength in two ways: either we can change the number of turns of the wire because more turns create more power, or we can put some kind of core inside the coil. An electric wire that has been coiled many times produces a field exactly like that of a bar magnet (see figure 4.1). As we create an electromagnet by putting iron or other materials inside the electric coils, a solenoid's magnetic strength will increase hundreds and thousands of times. Electromagnetic cores always used to be iron, but some cores are now ceramic, made from a non-metallic mineral such as clay. The human electromagnetic core may be the iron in hemoglobin and/or our clay-based cellular structures.

The power of electromagnets can be controlled by changing the number of turns of the coil, altering the core, and/or reversing the polarity. They can be turned off and on and they can be controlled from a distance by relays, which are weak electrical currents that open and close circuits in which a stronger current flows. Relays can be powered by electric currents as small as a millionth of an ampere.

The three-part human energetic anatomy acts like a sophisticated electrical and electromagnetic information processing system. Our bodies act like the hardware of a computer and our hemoglobin and clay-based cells may act as our electro-magnetic core. Chakras act like the software, the biofield stores the data, and the meridians act as if they carry data and provide the electrical power to control the system. All work together in ways not yet fully understood to send information throughout the organism.

## The Chakras

*Chakra* is a Sanskrit word for wheel or vortex of light. The human energy centers, or chakras (described in more detail in chapter 6) appear to be energy stations, receiving input from the unlimited supply of energy found in nature and releasing excess *Qi* when there is an overload. Figure 4.1 is a drawing of a simple electromagnet and magnetic field; imagine that it is also a picture of a single chakra as one might see it from above or below, placed on end. Figure 4.2 depicts an onion slice; as can be seen, an onion may be a simple model of a chakra's energetic structure.

If the root chakra, for example, functions as a solenoid, it might indeed look like an onion slice. The chakra's magnetic core would be deep within the body, perhaps in the spinal cord or in an even more subtle energy structure such as the *hara* energy line that is within or parallels the spinal cord. Recall that the power of a solenoid is determined by the number of electrical coils around its core. Leadbeater (1927) published beautiful color plates of the chakras, showing that

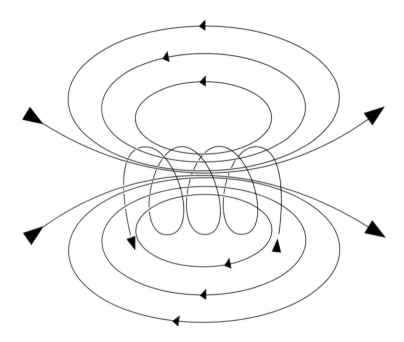

**FIGURE 4.1** A solenoid: note the core and field.

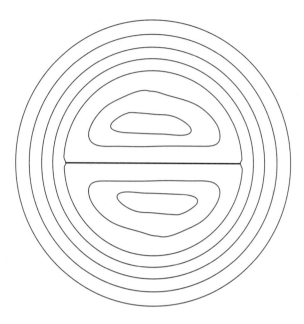

**FIGURE 4.2** A drawing of an onion slice that resembles a solenoid and its magnetic field

each succeeding chakra is more complex and has more sections than the one below. Chakra models, such as those offered by Brennan (1987), Bruyere (1989), Leadbeater (1927), Slater (2000), suggest that the root chakra processes the simplest data (survival), with each chakra in turn processing increasingly more complex information. For example, seventh chakra spiritual data is more complex than first chakra survival data. The simpler to increasingly more complex structure of the chakra chain resembles a series of solenoids of increasing power.

In figure 4.3, the magnetic field that surrounds an electrical current moves in a circle. Even though the magnetic field's movement is in the same horizontal, circular direction, one side of the field is moving in the opposite direction from the other side. The electrons moving through the coiled wire travel perpendicular to the magnetic field moving in the coil, thus the electrons will be moving in the same vertical direction with part of the magnetic field, and in the opposite direction of another part.

***Transformers as a Chakra Metaphor*** Transformers change electrical voltage and may offer a way to understand the sequential increase in power and complexity of the chakras. A solenoid of two coils is the simplest transformer. As described above, when the first coil is powered by an alternating current, it will induce an alternating current of the same frequency (wavelength) in a second coil. If the second coil has more turns of the wire than the first, the second coil will have a greater voltage; this is called a step-up transformer. If the second coil has fewer coils, the voltage will be less; this is a step-down transformer. There are

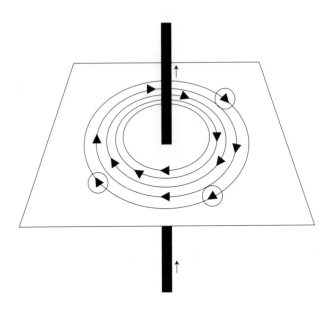

**FIGURE 4.3** A magnetic field surrounding an electrical wire

no moving parts in a transformer and the energy loss in a properly designed transformer is slight, often as low as 2% (Freeman, 1990, pp. 164–65).

Like step-up and step-down transformers, chakras amplify and/or reduce the electrical frequency in the chakra chain. As the root chakra receives the initial power, a current of the same frequency (wave length) is induced in the second chakra. Each chakra has unique functions, different than other chakras; otherwise, it would be like having each radio station receiving the same programs. Each chakra acts as if it is more complex and able to handle more energy than the one below it. As the first chakra induces an electrical flow in the second, the second increases, or steps up the power of that energy. The second chakra in turn induces a current in the more complex third chakra, and so on. The chakra chain acts like a transformer that incrementally steps up power through a series of increasingly complex solenoids.

Each chakra influences the more complex chakra above it, and the less complex chakra below it. A simultaneous step-up and step-down function may occur as each chakra influences the chakra above it and below it at the same time. The healing implications for this multidimensional image are stunning. For example, you might receive an impression through your root chakra—perhaps someone smiles at you when you believed that person didn't like you. This data courses through all of your charkas, disrupting and transforming the initial information that the person did not like you. When the new information reaches the heart chakra, you must deal with the task of giving a loving or non-loving response to this person; when it reaches the throat chakra, you must speak your own truth—"She likes me. Maybe she isn't so bad." That leads to an insight, "I misunderstood this person." As the sixth chakra, the intuitive center, is activated, it simultaneously activates the crown and the throat chakras. Your sixth chakra insight becomes a fifth chakra new truth, "I might want to get to know this person better," which transforms the data in each chakra in turn, until the ever-changing data gets back to the first chakra. The data has made a round trip and your chakra system once again faces the issue of survival and security, but you are able to view the world, or at least this person, differently. Thus, the whole action behaves like a simultaneous step-up and step-down process.

The round trip image illustrates only a portion of our actual energy flows. At the same time the energy is moving up the chakra chain, it is also moving down. For example, the energy of the fourth chakra transforms the fifth and third. By the time the new insight returns from its journey through the six and seventh chakras back to the third, it has already been transformed slightly by the series of changes in the fourth chakra. This multidirectional flow may explain why healing can occasionally occur so easily; it happens in baby steps but those steps are cumulative and transforming.

The HT technique Full Body Connection (described in chapter 10) seems to rely on this transformative function of chakras and takes advantage of the step-up transforming function of chakras. In this procedure the healer begins with the lowest chakras in the feet or ankles, and assists each "coil" to increase its power, which then radiates and flows to the next chakra, increasing its power, and so on up the chakra chain.

In chakras, the most crucial information of survival and safety is carried on lower frequency wavelengths that require a relatively simple system to process. Something is interpreted either as dangerous or not. The more sophisticated data, such as insights and spiritual wonder, require more powerful, faster wavelengths to hold the more complex information.

Chakras act like computers in their information processing functions. In computers, information is stored and carried on electromagnetic waves. The tiny gold wires on the hard drives and motherboards act like meridians; they carry the electrical current where it is needed. There are no moving parts in a computer, only moving electrons powered by a very small, thumbnail-sized battery. The data we enter is stored on an arrangement of electrons and their electromagnetic fields until it is needed again. The increasing power and capacity of computers is due to the ability to store more data in smaller spaces with higher frequency electromagnetic waves. Like a series of increasingly powerful computers, each chakra handles more energy, more complex tasks, and more complex information at faster speeds.

***Capacitors as Chakra Metaphors***    Chakras also act like capacitors, which store electricity up to their capacity until it is needed; the amount of electrical charge a battery can hold is called its electrical capacitance. An automotive battery is a series of capacitors that hold a charge for the duration of the battery's life. An electrical charge stored on a capacitor would flow to an area with fewer electrons if the capacitor were not insulated. This flow is called conduction. Typical insulators are made of glass, rubber, or even waxed paper. The relationship between a conductor of electrons and an insulator may illuminate the relationship between healer and client. When a conductor, such as a healer, is connected to an even larger object, such as the earth, it is said to be grounded. A grounded object will lose its charge either because the excess electrons will flow into the earth or the electrons needed to balance the charge will flow up from the earth. This may be part of the phenomenon of grounding; when the healer is properly grounded, any charge received from the client is simply discharged into the earth; if a charge is needed by the client, it may flow from the earth to the client.

When a charged object touches a conductor, the charge will spread over the entire surface of the conductor, which then becomes charged. Metals, such as gold and silver jewelry, are among the most efficient conductors. No one has reported measuring the charge on a healer's ring before and after a HT treatment, so the question of whether a healer should ground jewelry after a treatment remains unanswered.

Capacitors are essential in radios and televisions stations, which broadcast information through space to receivers. Receivers also use capacitors in detecting a signal. From the view of a chakra, this may be how one person picks up the energy/information from another person's chakras, how chakras send their information from one to another, and how healers broadcast energy to the client, with the healer's hands being the transmitting antennas.

Chakras act like solenoids, transformers, oscillators, and transmitters, receivers, and conductors, yet they do not have the elaborate electrical equipment that modern science has designed to do the same functions. While we don't know how chakras really are constructed, HT providers have sensed them often enough to know that they have physical properties: they have movement, they open and close, and they can be damaged. A person will frequently develop physical problems in the area of the body where a chakra is not functioning optimally. Each chakra is attributed with a specific task, as if it receives, processes, and transmits information on a particular frequency of light. Chakras appear to be exceedingly sophisticated data processing devices without the moving parts or structures that engineers have had to design. They also appear to act like semiconductors.

***Semiconductors and Transmission of Information***    Unlike conductors that carry energy from one place to another, or the wires that carry the electrical charge to your lamp, semiconductors are used to transmit and amplify electronic signals that contain information as well as energy. The best known use of semiconductors in our society is the computer. While the human body does not have the electronic devices within computers, still the computer and the human body function much the same. According to Oschman (1997), semiconductors

> . . .have the ability to *process* energy and information, i.e., to switch, store, delay, modulate, amplify, filter, detect, rectify (allow to pass in one direction but not in the other), etc. In addition, semiconductor networks can have read-only and programmable memory and logic circuits that evaluate the information flowing through them. In a living organism, such circuits could make and process decisions that lead to actions. The actions selected could be determined by a combination of genetic programming built into the circuitry, memory of previous activities, and current information from local and distant sources. (p. F-14)

Chakras have characteristics of semiconductors, but Oschman extends the semiconductor metaphor to include the entire body. He proposes that the collagen-rich connective tissue matrix and the meridians may make up a semiconducting electronic communication network. This tissue matrix may be the same as the bioelectric regulation system to which Rubik (1997) refers. If the tissue matrix is a semiconducting network, it may be how chakra information is transmitted from the chakra into nearby organs and other structures.

It has recently been discovered that all of the molecules in the body act as semiconductors enabling high-energy electrons to travel through the living human system much faster than is possible through neurons. Oschman (1997) writes:

> We now know that virtually all of the proteins in the body are semiconductors, and that the entire fabric of the body, including the smallest parts of cells, are semiconductors. This means the flexible living substance of which we are made is not only a structural material but is also an electronic communication network with the ability to detect and conduct energy and information, to store information, and to process signals. Wholeness, unity of structure and function, are natural consequences of having such a system within us. (p. G-4)

Oschman stresses the role of acupoints, but his description could also apply to chakras. Chakras and acupoints may act like individual microprocessing information nodes in which a very small local change will cause a change down the line. Oschman believes that many sources of information are integrated at these nodes, including data from the internal and external environments. The system may adjust for physical assaults, such as surgery or wounds, by rerouting the data flow. It may be like the Internet, which does not send your e-mail messages directly to you but through multiple sites. This indirect path permits continuing communication even if one avenue is blocked.

Semiconductors also allow energy to be converted from one form to another. In the human body, sound, heat, and tension, for example, can be converted into electrical energy and vice versa. Thus, an organism might hear a sound in the bushes. The sound may be converted into electrical energy by and rapidly transmitted through the chakra chain, permitting the individual to recognize if a noise represented a possible threat requiring a decision and action. A more complex and less instinctive response would be required if the noise were made by a child, a friend, or a complete stranger. As the data was rapidly processed and transformed up and down the chakra chain, our response would be a complex blend of data laid down through instinct, experiences, and choice.

Semiconductors fit the HT practitioners' experiences of healing through electrical and informational networks. If a practitioner senses that the network has been damaged because of surgery or physical or emotional trauma, she often will sense that the original flow has been "short circuited" and may be able to discern an alternate flow that bypasses the wound. The new flow may be less efficient than the original, but, like a distributed network, it enables the information and power to get where it is needed. Significant damage to the meridian-chakra distributed network may contribute to chronic fatigue and depression, which often lessen when chakra and meridian flows are repaired through clearing and rebalancing of a specific area.

## The Biofield

In the aura, or biofield, all of the information is contained in the electromagnetic wavelengths of light close to the surface of the body; each successive layer contains less dense information. Further from the surface of the body, some of the information becomes a whisper rather than a shout. If our information is carried on wavelengths of light, then our more abstract spiritual information is co-located with the physical information close to the surface of the body, but can only be "heard" after the lower frequency essentially has been muted. The auric information and structure is dynamic, it changes with each emotion and thought. Hunt (1981) found that its changes preceded verbal and nonverbal communication (p. 49).

The chakras and the biofield both appear to deal with data carried on different wavelengths of light. Chakras transform and conduct it; the aura may store it. Hunt (1995) measured the frequency of the aura as at least one million cycles per second, which is the speed of radio waves. At this speed, a cycle, one wavelength, is one kilometer long; visible light is made of smaller wavelengths that are between 10 microns (red) and 1 micron (violet) long. A human computer working at the speeds of visible light could store (in the aura) and process (via the chakras) a great deal of concrete and abstract information ranging from survival to wonder and more.

Benor (2000) studied multiple healers who were making intuitive diagnoses of the same person at the same time. Their impressions differed but the person being diagnosed found most of the information relevant. It was as if each healer focused on only part of the data available and understood only part of the total picture. The combined impressions provided a more complete and more accurate interpretation of the subject than any one of them. The two noted healers

Brennan and Kunz seem to have done this in their models of the biofield. Brennan (1987) noticed the differences inherent in data stored on a propagating, spreading electromagnetic field, while Kunz (1991) noticed the differences in the data being transformed and conducted from chakra to chakra. When the visions are combined, we get a picture of a matrix of data, as seen in chapter 5. Each aura/chakra aspect contains one permutation of the same information. Thus, the data at the auric layer closest to the body at the first chakra layer will be different from the data at the closest auric layer at the seventh chakra layer. Similarly, the data at the seventh auric layer at the first chakra will be different from the data at the seventh auric layer of the seventh chakra. This may explain why we keep revisiting our stories over and over, including the ones we think we have healed. We are processing the different permutations of the story in each of the data cells within our biofield/chakra matrix.

## Superconductors

The mechanism of superconductors may explain why some of our stories seem to have a life of their own, why we can't seem to process them and let them go easily. This phenomenon acts as if that data is carried on a superconductor. Superconductors are materials that conduct electric current without energy loss. In industry, superconductors can be created by keeping certain metals or some special ceramics at extremely low temperatures. In these conditions, those materials have zero resistance to electrical flow; there is no resistance and no diminution of power over time.

If a superconductor is in the shape of a ring and charged with electricity to get a current started, the current will continue to flow through the ring even after the charge is removed, a type of perpetual motion (Lindley, 1996). The fact that the current in a superconductor can last for years without loss of energy may be implicated in the incredible stability of emotional trauma. Even though we process and reprocess our grief, anger, hurt, and trauma, many of these feelings do not go away and may not even seem to diminish. Perhaps they are in a form of a superconductor "tape-loop." Perhaps one of the reasons energy healing rapidly helps to heal emotional wounds is that it provides an infusion of energy that disrupts the superconductor loop.

Superconductors may explain another human oddity—the ability to hold two contradictory opinions at the same time. If a small gap exists somewhere in a superconducting ring, it acts as a "weak link." If the gap is narrow, the current is able to jump the gap and continue to flow. The gap creates a lack of integrity in the ring, allowing the magnetic state inside to fluctuate, which in physics is described as jumping from one state to another. External magnetic fields can influence the ease with which such jumps can occur. It is as if both states exist simultaneously, or are superimposed, but external forces or chance determine which one will be active (Lindley, 1996).

There is an old adage that teenagers can think and feel, but do not do both at the same time. Any parent of teenagers is familiar with this phenomenon. One day, teenagers will carry on a remarkably rational and mature conversation about a problem and the next day lambast the world because it is set up wrong. As parents know, appeal to rational thinking is useless at these emotional times. Similarly, clients will believe two seemingly opposing truths, such as "I deserve to be loved, and I am unlovable." Perhaps HT treatments provide an energetic input that opens the gap in an emotional/mental superconductor-type system so that the two contradictory beliefs can be seen at the same time, reconciled, and integrated.

This section has shown how computer and electrical technology are useful metaphors to make the human energy system tangible, but any computer user knows that the computer is only a tool; it does not have a mind of its own. If no one intentionally chooses to operate a computer, it is a dust catcher taking up space on a desk. Our chakra/biofield/meridian computer acts on data for us, but it is not us. WE are more than our biological or electromagnetic data-filled structure. We act like the consciousness that pervades and operates it.

## THE POWER BEHIND HEALING TOUCH: CONSCIOUSNESS

Like the human energy system, our consciousness is another intangible human experience. The origin of consciousness is an ongoing debate. One school of thought is that consciousness emerges from biological processes, that it is a secondary phenomenon of molecular, physical, and physiological activities. In this view, consciousness is dependent on and determined by our biology. Another school of thought is that consciousness is independent of and precedes, even shapes, our biology (Sheldrake, 1981). Two images represent these contrasting views. One is that the body houses the mind/soul much as our cars contain us. The phrase "you are not your body" exemplifies this view. The other image is to see our consciousness and body as integral with each other; they look different and process data differently, but they are a unity. In this more complex view, you are your body, your mind, your emotions, and your spirit because they are one—and different—at the same time.

HT practitioners routinely experience the unity of body, mind, emotions, and spirit while giving HT treatments. As we work with a client, it becomes apparent that these are unitary aspects of the same phenomenon. Healing appears to occur electrically, magnetically, and consciously; it looks as if the hardware of the body needs time to respond to the changes in the wiring, the electromagnetic flow, and in the emotional and mental data. The power behind HT treatments and healing seems to be in the practitioner's and client's conscious intent and choice. The consciousness that HT practitioners and their clients encounter is transforming and transcendent, beyond our usual modes of understanding.

## Consciousness As the Only Reality

Physicist Fred Alan Wolf says, "[the] transcendental—outside of space-time, nonlocal, and all-pervading. It is the only reality..." (quoted in Goswami et al., 1995). The view that consciousness is the only reality is a minority but growing perspective in physics. Goswami suggests that, rather than everything being made of atoms as many scientists suggest, everything is made of consciousness. This radical view has emerged from some puzzling research findings. Quantum physics has discovered that an electron can be at more than one place at the same time (the wave property), but only becomes reality in one place when it is observed (collapse of the wave). Our observation of that quantum object influences its twin, no matter how far apart they are (quantum action-at-a-distance), and a quantum object can cease to exist here but appear somewhere else simultaneously (quantum jump) (Goswami et al., p. 9). Observations after the fact can determine how an electron will act in the past. The wave property is not a real wave, such as a water wave, but is a mathematically predicted wave like a crime wave.

Herbert (1985) has written one of the most lucid physics books for non-physicists, *Quantum Reality—Beyond the New Physics: An Excursion into Metaphysics and the Meaning of Reality*. He explains the eight quantum theories, which include the well-known theory that light is a wave and a particle at the same time, and the contradictory theories that reality is an undivided wholeness (the holographic theory) and many worlds (parallel worlds). He points out that eight incompatible quantum theories are experimentally indistinguishable, which suggests that there is an undiscovered phenomenon that connects them. Theorists suggest that the underlying phenomenon is consciousness. It is the observing device that selects which superimposed state in a superconductor will be active and which potential will collapse from a wave function into reality.

## Consciousness May Influence Reality: Intention

Some interesting research using random number generators suggests that consciousness may influence reality. Several research studies have been done to see if people deliberately and consciously influence the results of a random number generator (RNG) which is an electronic device that generates a series of odd and even numbers. Chance would assume that the odd and even numbers generated would be approximately the same, or 50/50. The question is, can randomness be made less random? Radin, Rebman, and Cross, who are with the University of Nevada Consciousness Research Laboratory, expanded upon studies showing that an individual can influence RNGs and tested the effects of group influence. They set up RNGs during two events: a day long Holotropic Breathwork session and the 67th Academy Awards broadcast. Twelve people were present in the Holotropic Breathwork class and 1 billion people in 120 countries were estimated to watch the 1995 Academy Awards broadcast. During the Holotropic Breathwork class, the RNG showed more order than was predicted during the times the group was engaged in a similar-focus, highly coherent task. During the lunch break and in the 9-hour control period, the RNG output behaved according to chance. Similarly, during the first half of the Academy Awards broadcast, there was a reduction in randomness, suggesting that "moments of *coherent attention* among one billion people introduced an anomalous degree of *order* into the environment" ( Radin, Rebman & Cross, 1996, p. 167). After checking with the Nielsen ratings, the researchers discovered that, as the audience gradually decreased throughout the ceremony, the degree of order decreased accordingly. The authors concluded that:

> (a) focused attention orders random events, (b) the effect of this ordering extends remotely, (c) the strength of the ordering effect increases when many individuals focus on the same object, even without explicit instructions to create order, and (d) the order is detectable as predictable fluctuations in the behavior of truly random events. (p. 167)

Gough and Shacklett (1993) define intention as "focused choice" (p. 198). The RNG studies suggest that if the client and healer are both focused on the same goal, it is more likely to occur. The problem is determining true mutual goals. While the healing practitioner is taught to have the intention that the healing is "for the client's highest good, in line with divine will, and with harm to none," the client may be visualizing his pain, hurt, grief, and misery. These are mixed visualizations, and, thus, mixed intentions. It might be useful for the client to hold thoughts of healing, but the healer cannot control another's thoughts and visualizations. It appears to be imperative that the healer maintain a clear vision of healing. Janet Mentgen teaches that Healing Touch is really the intention to communicate love, whether you are teaching HT or giving a HT treatment. Her thoughts have been echoed by other healers, including Mietek Wirkus, who, in 1987, told Dr. Benor, "You must love people, you cannot have any rancor, malice or hatred in you. Concentrating on kindness and love raises the energy level; it is a source of strength" ( Benor, 1992a, p. 45).

For optimum effectiveness, one must blend love with the intention to heal. Benor reported that many of the healers he interviewed maintain a simple intention: they hold a picture of a well person in their minds throughout the healing session. Lawrence LeShan (1976), who studied gifted healers, discovered that they visualized themselves united with the healee and with the "All."

Healers also may imagine or sense that *Qi* is flowing through them and trust that the clients will use it to their maximum benefit. Gordon Turner, whom Benor described as "one of this century's great English healers," wrote as follows:

I would . . . let my hands move lightly over the patient's body. As long as I could still my conscious mind they would be drawn to the exact spot where the treatment was needed. . . . it was essential that I avoided thinking about what my hands were doing . . . for that matter even looking at them. Healing had to be a spontaneous rather than an intellectual matter . . . If my attunement had been made too casually, or if I became too personally involved in the healing, it would be my own energy which was drawn upon. But if the attunement was good and my mind clear, I could feel the healing power flowing through me from some apparently inexhaustible source. On such occasions I could heal for hours without tiring. (Benor, 1992a, pp. 27–28)

## Healers' Traits and States

HT providers may fit Elaine Aron's (1997) description of highly sensitive people. She believes that 20% of the population have more highly sensitive nervous systems than others and an additional 20% have moderately sensitive systems. Highly and moderately sensitive nervous systems act like more finely-tuned radio receivers than less sensitive ones, and the trait may be hereditary. Highly sensitive people may have greater access to the information carried on the electromagnetic waves of light that surround us, but their use of that information is enhanced or hampered by how they have learned to use what they gather. If 60% to 80% of people discount the highly sensitive person's observations, many highly sensitive people will learn to distrust their impressions and tune them out. Those who have learned to trust what they perceive may be the "natural healers." The 60% of people with the least sensitive systems may not be able to sense energy easily and may be skeptics and opponents of energy therapies. The highly sensitive people may be those who gravitate toward Healing Touch and other energetic modalities; their learning to be healers may begin with their learning to listen to and trust the messages they receive.

## Centering

Centering may be a type of self-referencing biofeedback. Green (1995) describes learning how to self-regulate autonomic processes as "learning to relax and quiet the body, the emotions, and the mind, then imagining and visualizing what you want to have happen, 'feel' it happening, and then letting it happen, allowing the body to carry out the visualization" (p. 228).

Cooperstein's (1996) description of the experience of moving into an altered state of consciousness resembles an HT practitioner's and recipient's experience:

Nonordinary physical sensations may be experienced at this point, including "energy," "vibrations," rhythmic sensations and extraordinary heat or cold. Time distortions or a sense of timelessness is often reported.

Analytical and critical thinking is reduced and there is a sense of height-ened expectations. Verbal thinking decreases, sometimes to the point of "inner silence," and heightened emotional reactions are felt. The healer gains increased access to (normally) subconscious processes, resulting in sudden, information-bearing intuitions in the form of mental images, sym-bols or physical sensations. (p. 192)

Centering may involve controlling one's heart rate. Heart rate variability changes when the emotional state changes. Research has shown that when peo-ple shift their attention to their heart and feel love and appreciation, there is a greater balance between the sympathetic and parasympathetic nervous systems and their heart rates become coherent. When the person feels frustration, the heart rate increases in variability (McCraty, Atkinson, & Tiller, 1993). The inten-tion to feel compassion for one's client causes the heart, the strongest biomagnetic field in the body, to beat coherently. The probable effect on the body is an increased electromagnetic coherence, which may be related to the effects of self-referencing biofeedback. As one focuses one's intent on feeling empathy and visu-alizing healing, the heart rate becomes more coherent, the body and the brain waves follow suit. The coherent human may become a strong radiator of coher-ent electromagnetic radiation, which may influence the changes recipients expe-rience during healing. Such coherent individuals who were holding a beaker with DNA samples have been found to be able to alter the DNA shape, sometimes beyond that produced by temperature or other means that are known to influ-ence the shape of DNA (Gough, 1997).

***EEG studies of healers***    In 1969, Robert Beck studied the brain waves of heal-ers throughout the world. All of the healers tested produced similar low frequen-cy brain-wave patterns when they were healing in a centered state of conscious-ness (Oschman, 1997).

Other studies indicate that different healers enter different states during heal-ing, and it may have to do with their level of expertise. Sugano et al. (1994) found that the more expert healers had more changes in brain waves from baseline than the less experienced healers. Fahrion, Wirkus and Pooley (1992) found a higher and less variable synchrony of all the brain waves—beta, alpha, theta, and gamma—in the bioenergy practitioner than in the recipient, and it was highest and most stable during healing-at-a-distance. When they were in a centered state, Krieger and other TT practitioners produced rapid, synchronous beta brain waves between 13 and 32.75 Hz (Straneva, 2000, p. 7). Healers using other approaches had high amplitude alpha waves of 8–13 Hz and their right brain hemispheres were activated (Fahrion, Wirkus, & Pooley, 1992; Sugano, et al., 1994). In the alpha state, one is letting the mind wander, not thinking, alert but tranquil.

A recent study (Grinberg-Zylberbaum et al., 1992) has shown that the brain waves of people at a distance can change when someone else's brain waves change.

The ability to detect and respond to such changes may be part of our human heritage and part of the success of our survival as a species. Such group coherence would help the relatively weak human individual gather with others to collectively combat threats. Similarly, brain waves have been shown to change in concert with the healer's. Wilson (1993) studied a natural healer from New Zealand; the client's alpha brain waves changed toward the healer's brain-wave pattern and returned to baseline after the healing. Sugano et al. (1994) studied practitioners of *Qigong* and Medical Art of Japan (Jorei) and found that their recipients showed a synchronization of alpha waves with increased frontal lobe activity. This suggests that the changes in brain waves during healing cannot simply be due to increased drowsiness. Wilson (1993) states that "when we let go of alpha we go into a more immediate awareness of what is in this moment, not what we expect it to be" (p. 178). Perhaps when we drop our expectations, healing can occur; perhaps this is when the magnetic flux of our emotional superconductor rings can be more easily nudged into a new, emotionally healthier state.

The New Zealander whom Wilson studied showed no evidence of change in alpha, beta, or theta brain waves but had powerful high frequency brain waves. The healer's brain waves in the center of the head were 1–6 Hz (delta and theta), but his temporal brain waves were up to 128 Hz at 39 microvolts, which is very high and very powerful. The normal delta, theta, alpha, and beta brain waves are rarely more than 20 microvolts. As Wilson (1993) described it, "the temporal lobes alone were lit up" (p. 176). He concluded that the shift in consciousness into a healing state "is maintained by holding a very low-frequency/high-amplitude activity in one part of the brain, and then shifting power up into the temporal lobes" (p. 178). He found that people who have psychic activity or who channel but who cannot remember the content of their experiences have hyperactivity in the right temporal lobe only. Those who remember what occurred have hyperactivity in both right and left temporal lobes. While most of the research on healer's states of consciousness has focused on coherent brain waves, Wilson's results suggest that brain regionalization may also be involved.

While high neurological sensitivity and the ability hold a clear vision of healing may be the primary variables required for successful healing, they may not be the only factors involved. Recent discoveries about geomagnetic fluxes indicate they may also influence healing work. Extrasensory perception (ESP) such as clairvoyance appears to be more intense or more frequent during periods of subdued geomagnetic activity (Krippner & Persinger, 1996). Becker (1992) found magnetite particles in the pineal gland creating a magnetic-field sensing system. Other scientists found magnetite particles throughout the brain, but concentrated in the meninges (Upledger, 1999). Becker suggests that the human "magnetic sense" acts as a detector of the environmental electromagnetic field. Increased geomagnetic activity might interfere with the ability of the magnetic sense to accurately receive and interpret the data carried on this field. HT practitioners might find that on such days they are less in tune with their clients and may or may not find centering more difficult.

## SUMMARY

While little is known about how Healing Touch works, a combination of evidence gathered here suggests possible mechanisms. The body acts like an electromagnetic organism and an exceptionally sensitive electromagnetic sensing device. Geomagnetic activity, such as solar flares, interfere with the electromagnetic organism's ability to sense the electromagnetic field surrounding it. By concentrating on feeling love for the recipient, a HT practitioner may increase the coherence of his field and may increase his ability to detect the data carried on the recipient's electromagnetic field. When a healing intention is added to the feeling of love, the effect on the recipient may be increased hydrogen bonding and decreased surface tension of water, weakening of superconducting rings, and an increase in the capacitance of chakras, thus strengthening the electrical and magnetic system, changing the data within the system, and increasing the efficiency of metabolism. Perhaps, the increase in metabolic efficiency is why many clients' bladders fill up quickly during a HT treatment and there is often an increased appetite.

However, HT practitioners and clients know that these are only the superficial mechanisms and results of HT. The deep, deep healing of memories, emotions, tangled histories, physical problems, and spiritual pain that is characteristic of HT treatments may be supported by alterations in the chakra, meridians, the semiconductor network, and in the information carried on the aura, but the depth of healing associated with HT occurs at the soul level. Perhaps the true mechanism of HT cannot be touched by empirical science; it is the conscious choice of an individual who chooses to enter his or her entangled quantum data, untangle it, restructure it, and, essentially, go back into the past and change the configuration of the electronic data laid down years ago. That is healing and it is life-changing. Healing Touch practitioners see such healing regularly and our sense is that the energy provided by a coherent, love- and intention-filled, expert HT practitioner who visualizes healing for another enables that person to jumpstart his or her healing. The task of HT practitioners is to strengthen our own capacitors, heal our entangled emotional and mental histories, love ourselves, and love others. That's all. That appears to be the real mechanism behind HT.

## REFERENCES

Aron, E. N. (1997). *The highly sensitive person.* New York: Broadway Books.
Becker, R. O. (1992). Modern bioelectromagnetics & functions of the central nervous system. *Subtle Energies, 3* (1), 53–72.

Becker, R., & Selden, G. (1985). *The body electric: Electromagnetism and the foundation of life.* New York: William Morrow/Quill.

Benor, D. (1986). Intuitive diagnosis. *Subtle Energies, 3* (2), 41–64.

Benor, D. (1992a). *Healing research: Holistic energy medicine and spirituality.* Volume I, *Research in healing.* United Kingdom: Helix Press.

Benor, D. (1992b). *Healing research: Holistic energy medicine and spirituality.* Volume II, *Holistic energy medicine and the energy body.* United Kingdom: Helix Press.

Benor, D. (2000). *Spiritual healing.* Vol. 1–4. Springfield, MI: Vision Publications.

Bloomfield, L. A. (1997). *How things work: The physics of everyday life.* New York: John Wiley & Sons.

Brennan, B. A. (1987). *Hands of light: A guide to healing through the human energy field.* New York: Bantam Books.

Bruyere, R. L. (1989). *Wheels of light: A study of the chakras.* Sierra Madre, CA: Bon Publications.

Cooperstein, M. A. (1996). Consciousness and cognition in alternative healers: An interim report on research into the relationship of belief, healing, and purported subtle energies. *Subtle Energies 3* (7), 185–238.

Fahrion, S. L., Wirkus, M., & Pooley, P. (1992). EEG amplitude, brain mapping, & synchrony in and between a bioenergy practitioner & client during healing. *Subtle Energies 3* (1), 19– 52.

Freeman, I. M. (1990). *Physics made simple.* New York: Doubleday.

Gonick, L., & Huffman, A. (1990). *The cartoon guide to physics.* New York: HarperPerennial.

Goswami, A., Reed, R. E., & Goswami, M. (1995). *The self-aware universe. How consciousness creates the material world.* New York: J. P. Tarcher/Putnam.

Gough, W. C. (1997). The cellular communication process and alternative modes of healing. *Subtle Energies, 8*(2), 67–101.

Gough, W. C., & Shacklett, R. L. (1993). The science of connectiveness: Part III: The human experience. *Subtle Energies, 4* (3), 187–214.

Green, A. M. (1995). Biofeedback methodology in psychophysiologic self-regulation. *Subtle Energies, 6* (3), 227–240.

Green, J., & Shellenberger, R. (1993). The subtle energy of love. *Subtle Energies. 4* (3), 31-55.

Grinberg-Zylberbaum, J., Delaflor, M., Sanchez Arellano, M. E., Guevara, M. A., & Perez, M. (1992). Human communication and the electrophysiological activity of the brain. *Subtle Energies, 3* (3), 25–43.

Herbert, N. (1985). *Quantum reality: Beyond the new physics. An excursion into metaphysics and the meaning of reality.* New York: Doubleday.

Hunt, V. V. (1995). *Infinite mind: The science of human vibrations.* Malibu, CA: Malibu.

Hunt, V. (1981). Scientific research on psychic energies at the department of kinesiology, U.C.L.A. *The Journal of Holistic Health, 6,* 47–54.

Krippner, S., & Persinger, M. (1996). Enhanced congruence between dreams and distant target material during periods of decreased geomagnetic activity. *Journal of Scientific Exploration, 10* (4), 487-494.

Kunz, D. V. G. (1991). *The personal aura.* Wheaten, IL: Quest Books.

Leadbeater, C. W. (1927). *The chakras.* Wheaton, IL: Quest Books.

LeShan, L. (1976). *Alternate realities: The search for the full human being.* New York: Evans.

Lindley, D. (1996). *Where does the weirdness go? Why quantum mechanics is strange, but not as strange as you think.* New York: Basic Books.

McCraty, R., Atkinson, M., & Tiller, W. A. (1993). New electrophysiological correlates associated with intentional heart focus. *Subtle Energies, 4* (3), 251–268.

Motoyama, H. (1997). *Treatment principles of oriental medicine from an electrophysiological viewpoint.* Tokyo: Human Sciences Press.

Oschman, J. L. (1997). *Readings on the scientific basis of bodywork, energetic, and movement therapies.* Privately printed. Dover, NH: N.O.R.A.

Oschman, J. L. (2000). *Energy medicine: The scientific basis.* Edinburgh: Churchill Livingstone.

Radin, D. I., Rebman, J. M., & Cross, M. P. (1996). Anomalous organization of random events by group consciousness: Two exploratory experiments. *Journal of Scientific Exploration, 10* (1), 143–168.

Rubik, G. (1997). The unifying concept of information in acupuncture and other energy medicine modalities. *The Journal of Alternative and Complementary Medicine, 3,* Supplement 1, 67–76.

Sheldrake, R. (1981). *A new science of life: The hypothesis of formative causation.* Los Angeles: Jeremy P. Tarcher, Inc.

Slater, V. (1996). *Safety, elements, and the effect of HT on chronic, non-malignant abdominal pain.* Lakewood, CO: Healing Touch International Research Listing.

Slater, V. E. (2000). Energetic healing. In B. M. Dossey, L. Keegan, & C. E. Guzzetta (Eds.), *Holistic nursing: A handbook for practice* (3rd ed.). Gaithersburg, MD: Aspen. p.125-154.

Snyderman, R. (Sept., 2000). CAM and the role of the academic health center. *Alternative Therapies. 6* (5), 86–93.

Straneva, J. A. (2000). Therapeutic touch coming of age. *Holistic Nursing Practice, 14* (3), 1–13.

Sugano, H., Uchida, S. & Kuramoto, I. (1994). A new approach to the studies of subtle energies. *Subtle Energies, 5* (2), 143–166.

Wilson, E. S. (1993). The transits of consciousness. *Subtle Energies, 4* (2), 171–186.

Upledger, J. E. (April, 1999). The use and abuse of magnets in healthcare. *Journal of Bodywork and Movement Therapies, 3* (2), 67–73.

Zimmerman, J. (1990). Laying-on-of-hands healing and therapeutic touch: a testable theory. *BEMI Currents, Journal of the Bio-Electro-Magnetics Institute, 2* (8), 1–17. [Available from Dr. John Zimmerman, 2490 West Moana Lane, Reno, Nevada 89509-3936, USA.]

# CHAPTER 5

# Identified Aspects of the Human Energy System

*"The concept of 'field' provides a means of perceiving people and their respective evironments as irreducible wholes."*
—M. Rogers, 1970

*"The nerve cells in the human brain are sufficiently sensitive to register the absorption of a single photon."*
—D. Zohar in Oschman,1998

## INTRODUCTION

In this chapter we shall explore the three identified and most prominent aspects of the human energy system. We shall also explore possible theories and develop considerations for a practice of energy healing, such as the known practice of Healing Touch.

## SCIENTIFIC DEVELOPMENTS

The term "subtle energy" was first used by famed physicist Albert Einstein to describe the minute, ongoing interrelationships between subatomic particles. In his quest for a unified field theory, he posited that there is interaction between matter and energy: energy, the driving force that we observe in the known universe, is related to matter and a proposed constant, that he presumed to be the speed of light (the famous formula is $E=mc^2$). Translated into human terms, it appears that our vital life force, *Qi*, or *prana*, is the very stuff of the universe. This energy is in continuous interaction with matter, as exemplified by our physical bodies, and the speed of our thoughts augmented by our emotions and sensitivity to our highest potential.

The actual presence of subtle energies in relation to the human organism is being explored by a number of scientists, as the previous chapter indicates, and is supported by the ever more specific instrumentation that is becoming available. In the early 1960s, Dr. Robert Becker (1990), for example, began to explore the slight electrical circuitry in the human body in an attempt to understand non-union problems in complex bone fractures. Over the next thirty years, he mapped an energetic system that parallels the human nervous system, is electromagnetic in nature, and functions to inform all parts of the human organism (p. 80). He proposed that this dual information system—the dissectable aspects of the human nervous system (brain, nerves, plexi, and ganglions) and the subtle energy system consisting of electrical circuits, energy vortices, and the electromagnetic field—is a form of natural redundancy. That is to say, in case one or more aspects of either system do not function fully, other aspects can take over and allow interrelationships and information to flow in the human body. For example, a person who has suffered a severe stroke with total hemiplegia can still think, digest food, produce endorphins, and recover many functions over time.

In a different vein, Dr. Hiroshi Motoyama (1997), physicist and yoga master from Japan, has shown the reality of the electronic circuitry exemplified in meridians and acupoints. His most recent work includes refinement for public use of the AMI (Apparatus for Meridian Identification), a computer that analyzes information from electrodes placed on fingers and toes, to identify imbalance in each of the meridians and the related organs, as well as imbalance in the major energy centers. Imbalance in the entire electromagnetic system, including the field, is being studied as well in a copper-lined room that would prevent any external interference or electronic artifact (personal communications, California Institute of Human Sciences, Encinitas, CA, 2000).

Thus, we are beginning to have scientific evidence to support the presence of the subtle human energy system. Our understanding to this date is that there are three major aspects of this electromagnetic information processing system. As Dr. Slater states in the previous chapter, "Our bodies act like the hardware of a computer and our hemoglobin and clay-based cells may act as our electromagnetic core. Chakras act like the software, the biofield stores the data, and the meridians act as if they carry data and provide the electrical power to control the system (p. 44)."

As a whole, this three-fold subtle energy system is continuously interactive within itself and with all other human informational systems, such as blood circulation, lymph flows, chemical messengers, neural pathways. We might correctly say that these interactions are vibrational in nature. Vibratory patterns are evidenced in the human body and can be measured with current medical diagnostic tools. In fact, medicine is quickly becoming vibrational as scientific advances move forward at an ever-increasing pace (Gerber, 2001). Properties of the organism can be measured *electrically* (electrocardiogram, electroencephalogram); they can be measured *magnetically* (magnetocardiogram, magnetoencephalogram); they can be measured *acoustically* (crystallography, lighography), as well as *elastically* (spectroscopy) and *thermally* (photometry, thermographic imagery) (Oschman, 1998).

It is helpful, then, to think of each whole human being as a vast network of vibrational interrelationships supported by the complex, subtle circuitry suggested—it is, indeed, a vibrational matrix. This vibrational matrix, in our present knowledge, consists of three major aspects—the biofield, the chakras, and the meridians. Subsets of these aspects are also being defined, such as the "basic grid," the "Celtic weave," the "five rhythms," and the "strange flows" described in Donna Eden's (1998) valuable book *Energy Medicine*. We will explore each of the three major aspects and begin to show implications for healing practice.

## THE CHAKRAS

The word *chakra* means '"wheel" or "vortex" in Sanskrit, suggesting a whirling center of human *Qi*. The energy centers are sensed in relation to the midline and the human spine, from the base of the tailbone to the area above the top of the head (see figure 5.1). They are known in some form in all human cultures, having their roots in native healing traditions for thousands of years, long before written communication developed.

One of the gifts of the chakras to our modern world is that they relate directly to the human body and psyche and can be sensed in some way by even the most concrete thinkers, the 60% of the population Aron (1997) calls "insensitive."

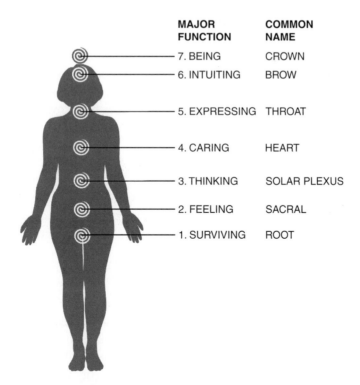

**FIGURE 5.1** Location of the 7 Major Energy Centers.

Thus, the chakras give access to deeper somatic and psychological awareness in persons who might otherwise reject personal intuition or self-care.

The physical, emotional, mental, and spiritual aspects of optimally functioning chakras are described in depth in the next chapter. Impaired, blocked, or diminished chakra function has profound effects on biological, emotional, mental, and spiritual health. Understanding this reality has direct implications for assessment and implementation of the healing interventions that will be defined more fully in the rest of this book.

The chakras seem to act like energy transfer stations. That is, they allow the inflow of *Qi* from the unlimited supply of energy in the Universe to enter the human organism; they allow this *Qi* to be dispersed throughout the individual's system; and they permit release, or outflow of excessive, unneeded, energy. Because work with the chakras is meaningful for physical as well as emotional healing, a developing trend is addressing the chakras in psychotherapy settings as a form of comprehensive energy psychology (Hover-Kramer & Shames, 1997; Grudermeyer & Hover-Kramer, 2000.)

## THE MERIDIANS

As already suggested, the 14 major meridians form the electromagnetic circuitry of the human body while hundreds of acupoints form the relay stations or boosters of these circuits. The practice of acupuncture, while known in China for over 5,000 years, did not become popular in the West until 1972. During the well-publicized first diplomatic trip to China, President Nixon's press secretary underwent an appendectomy without any anesthesia other than the use of acupuncture. Even more remarkable was the fact that he recovered more quickly than from surgery in the West, walking almost immediately and without after-effects from anesthesia.

It was only in 1997 that the American Medical Association (AMA) and the National Institutes of Health (NIH) officially acknowledged the benefits of acupuncture for the treatment of certain conditions like chronic pain and nausea (NIH, 1997). This has opened the door to many new ways of understanding mind/body interactions and developing integrative practices between traditional Western medicine and thinking in energetic terms.

Although Healing Touch practice does not specifically address work with the meridians, the premise that we are working with the subtle interactions of the human energy system is strong. Some Healing Touch practitioners combine their work with meridian approaches. Many new practices are emerging with specific meridian therapies that do not use needles to stimulate the acupoints. One of these is the work of acupressure; another is the work of energy psychology (Gallo, 1998; 2000). The emerging field of comprehensive energy psychology (resources listed in the Appendix) combines work with the biofield, the meridians, and the chakras to bring relief from psychological distress.

## THE BIOFIELD

In 1970, long before scientific documentation of subtle energies and the interconnectedness of human beings with their environments was available, nursing theorist Dr. Martha Rogers published her concepts of the human energy field in the *Science of Unitary Human Beings*. She described her ideas, based on extensive study of quantum physics, as follows:

> An energy field identifies the conceptual boundaries of man. This field is electrical in nature, is in a continual state of flux, and varies continuously in its intensity, density, and extent. . . the human field is postulated to have its boundary continuous with the boundary of the environment. The environment is, itself, an energy field electrical in nature. The interaction between the human field and the environmental field takes place across the conceptual boundaries of these two fields which together are co-extensive with the universe. (Rogers, 1970, p. 90)

Thus, we have, in the art and science of nursing, an early formulation of the irreducible nature of the human being as an energy field that is integral and interactive with other fields. This became the theoretical foundation of the use of non-invasive, energetic interventions to assist someone in need, someone in whom the energy field was impaired, blocked, or depleted. Dr. Dolores Krieger, later to be co-founder with Dora Kunz of Therapeutic Touch, was one of Dr. Rogers's students at New York University over thirty years ago. Together they posited that the nurse/patient relationship is a virtual interaction of two human fields—the field of the nurse and that of the client.

Fields bring objects separated by space into relation with each other. In the past hundred years, the term field to describe an invisible and nonmaterial emanation from an object has come into use in scientific terminology. For instance, the electromagnetic envelope generated by a dynamo is called its electromagnetic field. Increasing scientific evidence, especially from quantum mechanics, holds that all bodies, from the atom and subatomic particles to the great earth itself, have their own fields, whatever size they may be (Capra, 1977, p. 196).

More than a hundred years ago, the well-known British physicist Faraday saw with intuitive perception the lines of stress or "force fields" surrounding magnets, and used this perception to describe the action of electric currents in space (Capra, 1977, p. 47). Faraday also sensed that the entire universe is made up of these force field lines and perceived light as electromagnetic radiation long before science could prove the nature of light as wave and particle. What Faraday sensed at the intuitive level was later proven mathematically and empirically to be correct.

The animal kingdom makes good use of the reality of energy fields in stalking prey. Sharks and rays, for instance, have electroreceptors that aid them in finding future meals, as all living organisms emit electromagnetic vibrations and have an energy field. Recent findings suggest that some mammals also use electroreceptors in settings where vision is limited, as in the case of the burrowing "electric" mole (Zimmer, 1993, p. 16). It appears, then, that the energy field is a fundamental underlying unit of all matter and is especially prominent in living systems.

Moving up the evolutionary ladder, we can recognize that there is an energy field that surrounds, flows through, and extends from the human body. It is undoubtedly more complex than that of the animal kingdom and can be sensed with the development of our higher sense perceptions. In ancient times, this emanation was called the *aura* and was perceived by mystics and clairvoyants as a visible phenomenon. We are now able to measure this biofield, or human energy emanation, with delicate scientific instruments. The Japanese physicist Motoyama (1997) has developed a number of electrode devices that measure the human bioelectrical field at various distances from the surface of the body.

We can have increasing appreciation for the sensitives and clairvoyants who accurately described biofields long before scientific confirmation was available. With tools only of higher sense perception of subtle energies, clairvoyants like Dora Kunz (Karigulla & Kunz, 1989) were able to diagnose complex medical problems by sensing the client's energy and noting "fullness" or "emptiness" in relation to parts of the body. In his work as a physicist, Motoyama (1984) "found strong correlation between meridians that are electrically out of balance and the presence of underlying disease" (p. 257). Thus, it is now possible to clinically assess a person's energy field to determine where there is an excess or lack of energy as a way of learning about a client's state of health. *Vibrational Medicine* (Gerber, 2001) is a fascinating book that captures the essence of this new energy-based approach and its implications for medical practice.

It is not so much that we *have* an energy field but rather that we *are* an energy matrix of which the physical body is the most visible and dense. The field essentially remains the same, whereas the material "stuff" of which we are made is constantly changing. Like a river that is consistent in shape but ever changing in content, the human body changes its cellular and molecular structure daily. Linings of the intestinal tract change every 3 to 4 days; other tissues replace and repair themselves in a few weeks (Chopra, 1991, p. 48). We know the physical body to be more than 75% water, but even the molecules of water are 99.99% space as we understand the conclusions quantum physicists draw about the nature of the spaces between subatomic particles. Within the energy field, protein and water molecules vibrate synchronously to influence ganglia, nerve plexuses, blood composition, endocrine secretions, and a multitude of other body processes. Emotions and thoughts vibrate within the biofield as well and may serve to transmit feelings and information to other human beings.

# Layers of the Biofield

Let us move on now to the specific layers of the human energy field and how they create a new understanding of ourselves and what may occur during a healing session. Many texts, both ancient and modern, describe the various layers, sheaths, or bodies of the energy field (Kunz & Peper, 1985; Leadbeater, 1980).

***The Work of Dora Kunz***    For nursing and the healing professions, Dora Kunz is best known as the gentle and persistent influence behind Dr. Dolores Krieger's development of Therapeutic Touch at New York University. Together they pioneered the development of the first modern, energy-based therapy and brought their knowledge to students throughout the world. Although many texts discuss the possibility of seven or more layers in the energy field, for our discussion we will use Kunz's four-level description. Her framework gives many insights about functions of the field layers and implications for assessment and intervention.

According to Kunz, these are the four major layers or dimensions of the energy field of most direct significance for healing work (Kunz & Peper, 1985, pp. 213–261):

1. The vital layer, also sometimes called the *etheric field*, is most closely associated with the physical body and interfaces with the emotional dimension. It extends 2 to 12 inches from the skin and is the layer most associated with energy-balancing healing work.

2. The emotional layer, sometimes loosely called *aura* in older texts, extends further than the etheric field, and holds the individual's affective, feeling energy.

3. The mental layer, still further from the skin, embodies our thinking patterns and visual imagery. It is often called the *causal layer* in ancient texts.

4. The intuitive layer, sometimes called the *astral body* in metaphysics, relates to the spiritual dimension of the individual.

Other layers of the energy field that have been observed are the etheric template, the celestial body, and the ketheric body, which constitute the physical, emotional, and mental aspects in the more subtle planes (Brennan, 1987, p. 47). See figure 5.2

***Sensing the Biofield***    As the energy field of the client is sensed, the practitioner can assess the state of the biofield. Lowered energy in the vital field, for example, is often the precursor of physical pathology. This state may be experienced by the client as irritability or fatigue. Often, field assessment with the hands can detect dysfunction before it actually becomes physical illness or more severe exhaustion. This suggests the great value of energy-based modalities in giving early feedback before symptoms become evident in the physical body. The abili-

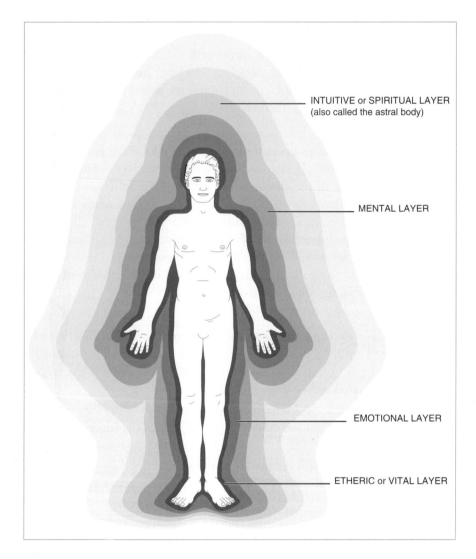

INTUITIVE or SPIRITUAL LAYER
(also called the astral body)

MENTAL LAYER

EMOTIONAL LAYER

ETHERIC or VITAL LAYER

**FIGURE 5.2** Four major layers of the human energy field extending beyond the physical body (other layers are also seen but are more subtle)

ty to detect impairments for early screening and prevention is thus one of the greatest gifts of the energy therapies.

## PRACTICAL APPLICATIONS

The recognition of the human being as a multidimensional field with energy as its dynamic force holds many implications for healing work. The mechanistic view of the body as a machine with replaceable parts gives way to the vision of each of us as a total human being who is at all times interconnected with the environment. Each human interaction now can be viewed as an exchange of energy between two interacting fields, as figure 5.3 shows. From this image we can appreciate the need to approach the energy field of a client with care and awareness.

Another concern is awareness of our own field as caregivers. With practice and intentionality we can learn to be sensitive to areas of depletion or imbalance and learn how to remain in the best possible state of health. When we see the impact of the two energy fields on each other, we know there is no way to hide our internal state in the physical, emotional, mental, or spiritual dimensions. At best, therapists or healers can recognize that their attitudes, beliefs, and opinions are communicated in many, often subliminal, ways. As psychotherapists have come to recognize, communication is a multilevel process, and we may not even know which part of our subconscious qualities reaches the subconscious of the client (Bandler & Grinder, 1975). Increasing our self-awareness and self-healing capacity is, therefore, our most important goal. This will be explored in depth in the last part of the book.

## Working with the BioField Layers

As we look at the client, we come to see that imbalance or dysfunction may occur in any of the layers of the energy field. To use the four-dimensional pattern

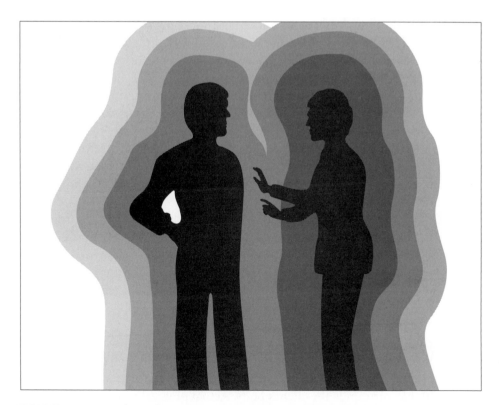

**FIGURE 5.3** Human interaction seen as an energy exchange of the two fields.

seen in figure 5.2, we note that each successive layer encompasses more of the whole than the previous one, although they are probably not as separate or discrete as the diagram suggests. Seeing the layers of the energy field also shows us the reasons that removal of a physical problem, as by surgical procedure, is often not sufficient to bring balance and harmony to the entire system. To put it another way, the body is influenced by the emotions, the mind, and the spiritual consciousness of the individual. The mind, connected to Infinite Intelligence, is much more complex than the body, the emotions, or thoughts by themselves, and encompasses or enfolds all of them.

As we see the model of the successive layers of the energy field, we observe that dysfunction in the spiritual, or intuitive, layer is undoubtedly the most devastating because it impacts all other layers. It is no accident that the great psychologist, Carl Jung, declared that the most significant disease of the twentieth century is loss of meaning and spiritual disconnection (Jung, 1964). Dysfunction in the spiritual layer is experienced as a loss of purpose or sense of hope in one's life. Dysfunction in the mental layer is manifest in faulty thought patterns and self-doubt. Dysfunction in the emotional layer relates to constricting affect, such as depression or despair. Dysfunction or blockage of energy flows in the physical dimension, and the related vital layer, can result in physical symptoms and disease over time.

This way of thinking leads us to understand most physical disease as the end stage of a much longer process. Recent exploration into the adult onset of cancer, for example, suggests that the actual tumor development occurs within 1 to 3 years after a significant loss or shock (Simonton, Mathews-Simonton, & Creighton, 1981, pp. 47–64). Initially, the individual loses a sense of purpose or meaning in life. The world around the other person no longer seems friendly or hope-inspiring. Then, negative thought patterns begin to take form and predominate, such as "I can't make it" or "life is not worth living." In time, depression and other negative emotions take over. The dysfunction in the three outer layers may be present, then, prior to the onset at the cellular level of a progressive disease such as cancer.

Another way that physical problems develop quickly is by traumatic injury. It is important to remember that all the layers are affected, that the entire energy field is jarred by trauma or accident, not just the vital layer. Treatment, similar to the long-term disease process, requires working from the innermost layer of the field to the outer layers. In the case of surgical intervention, a rebalancing of all the layers of the field is needed to complete the healing process, as we shall explore in chapters on healing interventions.

Healing Touch is an easily learned approach that allows the practitioner to recognize deficiencies in the biofield of the client and to facilitate balance. As in all healing practices, the healer reaches out from the vital life force within herself to the biofield that surrounds the client's body. Actual physical touch does not seem to be important for balancing the biofield. Instead, the practitioner assesses the field and uses rhythmic hand movements to smooth a turbulent or congested area. This may be followed by holding the hands over the area to allow rebalancing and integration within the entire biofield to occur. We will consider these practices in more detail in chapter 8.

The exact dynamic of this approach to healing is not yet fully understood, but, as we saw in chapter 3, the effects of *Qi*-based healing interactions are measurable and significant. Application of these concepts in counseling work also shows that significant emotional changes can be effected by working directly with the human vibrational matrix. This will be described in more detail in chapter 15.

## Alignment with Higher Power

Another important implication of energy theory for the healer is alignment with our Higher Power as we may sense the unlimited supply of order and flow within nature. Barbara Brennan (1987), who began her appreciation of biofields as an astrophysicist looking at earth's magnetosphere in spacecraft images, calls this manifestation of the infinite the Universal Energy Field. The healer does not drain his own strengths and resources to help someone else. Rather, he is a conduit for the universal life energy, the Source, or Higher Power. Burnout among healers is not possible if we are continually tapping into this limitless energy supply via our centering work. A sense of feeling drained or exhausted suggests that the healer may be attempting to use her own ego power instead of trusting the universal flow. *Qi* seems to move or resonate from the person with more *Qi* to the person with depleted flow, from the stronger vibration to the weaker vibration, and to move the diminished pattern to a higher frequency. Therefore, it is essential that the healer be attuned to the higher vibrational frequencies and release as much personal tension or negativity as possible before reaching out to others.

## SUMMARY

In essence, then, an energy-based, noninvasive approach such as Healing Touch is the application of the principles of *Qi* balancing to the multidimensional field of the client. It appears there is a flow of energy from the Universal Energy Field through the healer to the client. To put it succinctly in computer language, there is input from the Universal Field, throughput of energy within the healer, and output to the client. The resonance that occurs in the interacting fields creates significant outcomes, bringing about changes in the physical, emotional, mental, and spiritual dimensions as we will explore in succeeding chapters. In addition, we will consider the individual energy centers and their relevance to multidimensional healing in the next chapter.

# REFERENCES

Aron, E. N. (1997). *The highly sensitive person*. New York: Broadway Books.

Bandler, R., & Grinder, J. (1975). *Patterns of the hypnotic techniques of Milton Erickson* (Vol. 1). Cupertino, CA: Meta Publications.

Becker, R. O. (1990). *Cross currents: The perils of electropollution, the promise of electromedicine*. New York: Tarcher/Putnam.

Brennan, B. (1987). *Hands of light*. New York: Bantam Books.

Capra, F. (1977). *The Tao of physics*. New York: Bantam Books.

Chopra, D. (1990). *Quantum healing*. New York: Bantam Books.

Eden, D. (1998). *Energy medicine*. New York: Tarcher/Putnam.

Gallo, F. P. (1998). *Energy psychology*. Boca Raton, FL: CRC Press.

Gallo, F. P. (2000). *Energy diagnostic and treatment methods*. New York: W. W. Norton & Co.

Gerber, R. (2001). *Vibrational medicine*. Rochester, VT: Bear and Co.

Grudermeyer, D., Grudermeyer, R., & Hover-Kramer D. (2000). *Individualized energy psychology: Training manual level II*. DelMar, CA: Willingness Works Press.

Hover-Kramer, D. & Shames, K. H. (1997). *Energetic approaches to emotional healing*. Albany, NY: Delmar.

Jung, C. G. (1964). *Man and his symbols*. New York: Doubleday and Co.

Karigulla, S., & Kunz, D. (1989). *The chakras and the human energy fields*. Wheaton, IL: Theosophical Publishing House.

Kunz, D., & Peper, E. (1985). Fields and their clinical implications. In D. Kunz, (Ed.), *Spiritual aspects of the healing arts*. Wheaton, IL: Theosophical Publishing House.

Leadbeater, C. W. (1980). *The chakras*. Wheaton, IL: Theosophical Publishing House. (Original work published in 1927)

Motoyama, H. (1984). *Theories of the chakras*. Wheaton, IL: Theosophical Publishing House.

Motoyama, H. (1997). *Treatment principles of oriental medicine from an electrophysiological viewpoint*. Tokyo: Human Sciences Press.

NIH Consensus Development Panel. (Nov., 1997). Acupuncture. *JAMA, 280*, 1518–1524.

Oschman, J. (1998). *What is healing energy? The scientific basis of energy medicine*. (originally published in *Journal of Bodywork and Movement Therapy* 1996–1998). New York: Churchill Livingstone.

Rogers, M. E. (1970). *The science of unitary human beings: An introduction to the theoretical basis of nursing*. Philadelphia: Davis Publishing Co.

Rogers, M. E. (1991). Nursing science and the space age. *Nursing Science Quarterly, 5* (1), 27–34.

Simonton, C., Mathews-Simonton, S., & Creighton, J. L. (1981). *Getting well again*. New York: Bantam Books.

Watson, J. (1985). *Nursing: The philosophy and science of caring*. Boulder, CO: Colorado Associated University Press.

Watson, J. (1988). *Nursing: Human science and human care.* New York: National League for Nursing.

Zimmer, C. (1993, August). The electric mole. *Discover Magazine.*

# CHAPTER 6

# The Chakras
# and Their Functions

> *"If one is to explore the world of inner experiences, his thoughts, his emotions and learn about himself, he must have some framework in which to do this. He must have a 'playroom' — a sort of workshop or laboratory in which he can experiment. . . . The framework provided by understanding the centers of consciousness (chakras) gives him a place to do this. It provides the student with a structured inner space in which he can play."*
>
> —Rama, Ballentine, & Ajaya, 1981

## INTRODUCTION

As we have seen, the human being is made up of a wondrous complex of layers or sheaths, starting with the physical body as the densest part and extending outward to form the dimensions of the entire biofield. Now we turn to another facet of the field, the concentrations or vortices of energy. They are called *chakras*, from the Sanskrit word for wheel. These points of focus for energy were seen by the ancients as vortices of color and light, spinning at various speeds and influencing the entire field. Thus, they were appropriately named *wheels of light*. In ancient as well as modern times, the chakras are understood as the receptors for the inflow of *Qi* from the Universal Energy Field and the gateways to consciousness. They appear to mediate communication between the various layers of the field and to ensure that energy flows to all parts of the human vibrational matrix.

## THE CHAKRAS

Many writings describe the chakras, from Hindu and Sanskrit texts that form part of yogic practices (Tansley, 1985) to the lovely clairvoyant visions of the American theosophists of the early twentieth century (Besant & Leadbeater, 1925). The great sleeping prophet, Edgar Cayce, described the energy vortices and their relation to physical ailments, giving specific cures for each dysfunction that was presented to him (Reilly & Brod, 1975). More recently, the work of transpersonal psychotherapists incorporates chakra theory into psychological awareness. And, to top off a large array of references, we have the dynamic, fully illustrated writings of Rosalyn Bruyere (1989) and Barbara Brennan (1987). (See also Slater, 2000; Judith, 1996; Eden, 1998)

Most of the material provides consensual agreement that the chakras exist and significantly influence the physical body as well as the emotions, mental patterns, and spiritual awareness. However, a great deal of diversity exists about specific facts, such as the particular functions of the physical body that are related to each chakra. Therefore, we are choosing for this discussion to follow the classical interpretation of Alice Bailey (1978, p. 45). Her work, which has been known for 50 years now, makes a definitive statement about complex body-mind interactions, and perhaps best exemplifies the cross-cultural orientation that is needed to comprehend the chakra system.

Many other smaller energy centers exist and are called minor chakras. For the present, we will concentrate on the seven major centers and their fascinating impact on our human vibrational matrix.

# LOCATION AND FUNCTION OF THE CHAKRAS

The following exploration of the chakras and their relationship to the biofield is based on extensive reading and the author's personal experience of working with the energy centers for more than 20 years. We will discuss the relation of each energy center to the body, to specific physiological functions, and to its influence on the endocrine glands. We will also consider the impact of the chakras in the psychological, mental, and spiritual dimensions to learn of the complex interrelationships that occur within the energy system. Table 6.1 will help in understanding the actual location of each energy vortex and its relation to the spinal column in the physical dimension of the energy field. Figure 5.1 in the previous chapter also gives the location of each center.

## The Root or Coccygeal Chakra

The root or base chakra is located at the base of the spine and radiates downward from the perineal area of the body. Its location below the coccyx gives it the name most frequently used. In the yogic tradition it is the *muladhara*, the manifestation of vital life energy. The color of bright, clear red is associated with the relatively slow vibration of this center, and a bumblebee captures its sound.

This center is related to the lower parts of the body — feet, legs, hips — and to functions of elimination and movement. Psychologically, this center is most related to our sense of belonging on the earth, feeling a sense of security, and having the will to survive and be fully alive. The adrenal glands, which sit on top of the kidneys, most influence this center through the body's survival responses. The

| TABLE 6.1 | The Seven Major Energy Centers | | |
|---|---|---|---|
| Location | Physical Area of Influence | Major Psychological Function | Color Vibrational Pattern |
| **Root** base of spine | Feet, legs, hips, perineum, adrenals | Connecting to survival, safety, vitality, joy | Red |
| **Sacral** below umbilicus & at sacrum | Lower abdomen, pelvis, gonads, assimilation & releasing | Feeling, letting emotions act as sensors, choosing, sexuality | Orange |
| **Solar Plexus** | Upper abdomen, early digestion, insulin production | Thinking, sense of power, identity, control, self-exsteem | Yellow |
| **Heart** | Circulation, heart, lymph flow, thymus | Caring, unconditional acceptance, & forgiveness | Green |
| **Throat** | Neck, voice, throat, thyroid | Expressing, creativity, humor, singing, writing | Light blue |
| **Brow** | Face, eyes, ears, pituitary | Seeing clearly, insight, intuition, & clairvoyance | Indigo blue |
| **Crown** top of head | Brain, biorhythms, pineal gland | Being, connecting to spirit, alignment with Higher Will | Purple, lavender, white to silver |

fight/flight reaction, stimulated by adrenal excitation, is the body's animal-like ability to generate physiological peak performance to ensure survival. Physiological and psychological distress generating fear and worry can constrict the energy of this center. The long-term stresses of our society, in which the adrenals are constantly agitated, can cause immeasurable physical and emotional damage as can be seen in functional hypertension and chronic anxiety states.

The will to live and to enjoy life is one of the greatest signs of optimum functioning of this chakra. As the body and mind are in close connection with each other, affirming mental patterns expand the energy flow through this center. Examples of life-affirming thoughts are "I feel my energy," "I am glad I am alive," "I am safe and secure; the universe is friendly." The related emotions are a sense of vitality, enthusiasm, and joy. The natural capacity to dance and move are physical expressions of this center.

## The Sacral Chakra

The sacral chakra, sometimes called the spleen center in ancient texts, is located halfway between the base of the spine and the end of the sternum, or just below the umbilicus. In the Indian texts this *svadhisthana* chakra is also related to the vital body energy and life force. The gonads, the endocrine glands of sexuality and reproduction, are associated with this center. Other related bodily functions are balance and assimilation of body fluids and absorption of nutrients through the large intestines.

Psychologically, this center is related to expressions of sexuality and the choosing of appropriate relationships. Most of the addictive processes that so plague our culture appear to have their origins in this chakra and rob it of its vitality. Many addictions, we are now learning, are actually caused by poor chemical assimilation of foods that, in turn, impacts other layers of the energy field. For instance, the long-term effects of chemical imbalance in the physical field can cause irritability and create the wish to escape the intensity of physical emotional pain. The pain can further be numbed by using addictive chemicals. Emotional imbalance and faulty thinking patterns develop over time to justify or rationalize this escape mechanism and become evident in other layers of the field as blocks in the flow of the *Qi*.

The color that exemplifies the sacral center is orange, and the melody of a wooden flute evokes its sound. Seeing options, making choices, and being responsible for one's actions characterize healthy functioning of the center. Emotional qualities include the abililty to use all of one's resources and available energies appropriately. In the mental layer of the energy field, this center enables us to discriminate between helpful and unhelpful influences and to release unwanted thoughts and ideas. When the center is activated in positive ways, relationships with others fall into place easily, and we are able to readily utilize and integrate new information.

## The Solar Plexus Chakra

Also called the *manipura*, this chakra is associated with power, strength, and the ability to feel one's ego identity. It is located near the solar plexus at the base of the sternum. The pancreas functions in this area by assisting in the digestion and storage of glucose. Physical distress, such as stomach ulcers, hypo- and hyperglycemia, and digestive disturbances of various kinds can be traced to blockage in the field around the third chakra.

Emotionally, this center relates to issues of control. People who have strong ego demands and dominate others represent an imbalance or distortion of this chakra. On the other hand, persons who are unduly passive or, worse yet, passive-aggressive, also demonstrate imbalance of this center. Healthy psychological manifestation of this center is in assertive behavior. The words that best express these patterns are "I trust my ability to communicate," "I communicate effectively," "I feel my strength and respect others' strengths." As this center relates to the ability to use ego awareness and intellect effectively, it represents the will to think.

The color of the solar plexus chakra is the one that literally aids mental functioning—clear, lemon yellow. The sweet sound of stringed instruments represents the musical essence. Esoteric literature reports this center to be a storage battery for extra energy to use in difficult times. It is the center associated with staying power, the ability to start things and bring them to completion. Masculine and feminine aspects within each of us are balanced and harmonized through the ability to give and to receive, which has its power in the solar plexus chakra.

## The Heart Chakra

The heart chakra, also called the *anahata* in the Indian tradition, is located at the center of the chest, between the nipples. The qualities of the heart center are those of harmonizing, loving, accepting love, and forgiving. The energy conveyed by this center is markedly different from that of the lower three that deal with the more material, earthbound work of ensuring survival, dealing with emotions, and thinking clearly. To put it another way, the lower centers address the physical, emotional, and mental dimensions as exemplified in the will to live, the will to feel, and the will to think. The heart center speaks from our soul level and is therefore associated with the will to love and accept ourselves and others.

The color of life and hope, emerald green, is related to this center, and it is often described as the transformative center. The radiating sound of bells gives the auditory vibration of the heart center's energy. It serves to mitigate the earthbound energies of the lower three centers with the subtle, higher centers of the spiritual or intuitive dimensions. The thymus gland, a small endocrine gland now understood as a major aspect of the immune system, relates to the physical dimension of this center. Associated physiological functions are the respiratory system and all parts of the cardiovascular network.

Heart center dysfunctions are plentiful at this time in history as heart disease and circulatory disorders are the leading cause of death in the West. The second leading cause of death is immune system dysfunction, either deficiency as in cancer and AIDS or overactivity as seen in the autoimmune diseases.

The heart is the seat of emotions we describe as love although we need to be careful to distinguish the kind of love we are discussing. Many popular song lyrics espouse a possessive emotion, more like the addiction and control of the second and third chakra areas, as love. The love of the heart center is a pure, spiritual caring, the essence of the thirteenth chapter of 1 Corinthians, verses 4, 5, 7, and 8 in the Bible: "Love is patient and kind; love is not jealous, or conceited, or proud;

love is not ill-mannered, or selfish, or irritable; love never gives up: its faith, hope and patience never fail. Love is eternal." In short, the heart represents unconditional acceptance and forgiveness.

When psychological work is done to release grudges, old hurts, and to forgive others, the energy of this center expands, which causes our immune system to become more active. Thought patterns for this center are "I forgive others easily," "I can give and receive unconditional positive regard," "I am loved and accepted by Universal Love." When we operate from the heart center and express devotion and service without internal conflicts, our true spiritual selves begin to emerge.

## The Throat Chakra

The throat center is located in relation to the middle of the neck and influences the thyroid gland. In the yoga tradition, the *vishuddha* is the center of creative energy. As its location suggests, it relates to the throat, neck, esophagus, and the function of making sounds by singing or speaking. Perceptions of the senses, communication, self-expression, and beginning intuitive awareness emanate from this center.

Those who have activated the throat center with the full support of the lower centers speak in a rich, sure tone of voice and enjoy expressing themselves in written and spoken communication, delighting in the sharing of ideas. Dysfunctions of the center are evidenced by constrictions of the voice, hoarseness, frogs in the throat, and the holding back of creative ideas. Poor self-image is another manifestation of fifth center blockage. When we believe others always know more than we do, there can be no sense of trust in ourselves or self-esteem.

The colors of turquoise or light blue express the vibration of the throat center as well as the sound of wind blowing through the trees. Clairaudience, the ability to hear intuitively, begins to emerge when this center is open. The capabilities associated with this chakra are the communication of one's talents, knowledge, and understanding, affirming "I enjoy expressing who I am." Needless to say, it takes a commitment to personal growth over many years to achieve the sense of purpose that is exemplified by the will to express oneself confidently.

## The Brow Chakra

As we continue to explore the finer, more subtle energies of the higher centers, we come to the brow chakra, often called the *ajna* center or the seat of the "third eye." Located in the middle of the forehead, this center is associated with the pituitary or master endocrine gland and is the focus of insight, vision, psychic awareness, clairvoyance, sentience, and the ability to sense nonphysical realities such as energy fields or auras.

As we might deduct, this center relates to the brain, eyes, ears, head, and nose in the physical dimension. Higher level thinking, mental processing, and sensory perception are other concomitants. In the emotional dimension, this center relates to a sense of self-identity, personal insight, and compassion for others. Mentally, when this center is active and open, there is a quality of knowing with wisdom, as opposed to mere cognition. The individual can evaluate and perceive accurately without judgment or prejudice, and unusual events are understandable from this expanded perspective.

Deep indigo blue is the color most often connected to this chakra and its sound is that of waves crashing on the beach. Increased ability to visualize and to receive mental imagery comes to us when this center is open and flowing. The willingness to see with insight and intuition or to put oneself in another's place characterizes this center. Another quality is the ability to combine unconditional love with wisdom.

Distortions of this center occur when a person taps into its perceptions without the grounding of the other centers. This is evidenced in the many persons who may have insights but use the information for selfish purposes or take a part of their experience to represent "the path" and impose it on themselves or others. Judgments and prejudicial thinking are another distortion of this level of consciousness.

## The Crown Chakra

The crown chakra, the *sahasrara* center, is located above the middle of the head where the fontanels are joined. It is understood as the spiritual center, the center of connection with the wisdom and oneness of the universe. The colors associated are white, orchid, lavender, or purple according to different traditions. The sound that best symbolizes this center is the universal, harmonizing tone of "om" or "aum." The center may also be understood as the unifying principle of all color into white and of all sounds into the rainbow of full orchestral music.

As this is the highest energy vortex in relation to the physical body, it is the center of spirituality and soul-consciousness. Love, openness, a sense of purpose and expansion beyond the ego personality, and alignment with Higher Power are the qualities of this center. The will to be and the will to do whatever is for the highest good are manifest through the open crown chakra. In many traditions, headdresses, crowns, and halos signify the person who is actively using this center to give spiritual leadership to others. Another beautiful symbol is the thousand-petaled lotus that gives an image of divine beauty and complex simplicity. Often, when a person feels the energy of this center, there is a unitive glimpse, a sense of oneness and interconnectedness with all creation, and a brief understanding of ways in which everything is unified and whole.

The pineal gland, which sits just above the pituitary, is the endocrine gland associated with the crown center. The actual physiological functions of this gland are being researched and appear to be related to the sense of timing that guides diurnal patterns, biorhythms, bodily functions such as the onset of puberty, and our responses to the seasons and sunlight (Tamarkin, Baird, & Almeida, 1985, p. 714; Liberman, 1991).

Seen as the seat of the soul, the crown center has no major dysfunctions since we are always in connection with the Source of Life. We may at times limit the inflow of vital energy from the Universal Energy Field by our limited thinking or blockage in the emotional or physical energy flows of the other centers. The words that capture the essence of the crown chakra are "I am whole," "I am one with the universe," and "We are all interconnected."

Some sensitives attuned to higher sense perception report the presence of chakras above the crown. These may be considered extensions of the crown chakra that connect us more actively with nonlocal aspects of ourselves. As we tap into the dimensions beyond our personal selves, the transpersonal or more-than-personal aspect is activated. This seems to be our human interface with the wider, more expanded dimension of consciousness that is currently being explored in the field of transpersonal psychology.

# RELATIONSHIP OF THE CHAKRAS TO THE BIOFIELD

In addressing the complexities of the chakra system, we are given an extraordinary and powerful tool for understanding human nature. We may wish to view the whole system as a useful metaphor for systematically tracking various aspects of body, emotions, mind, and spirit. Figure 6.1 helps us to visualize the chakras as they are felt: cone-shaped wheels of energy extending from their locations near the spinal column through the ever finer layers of the energy field, in both the front and back of the body.

As we combine the various qualities of each chakra and its relationship to the four major layers of the energy field, we can imagine a comprehensive chart, as in table 6.2, to show the optimum functioning of each chakra. Knowing the optimum functions allows us in the healing professions to spot deviations that could indicate early stages of dysfunction. We will also be able to make comparisons between relative states of wellness and the various dysfunctions to identify areas for healing work.

If we summarize the dysfunctions in relation to each center, we can trace the impact of imbalance on the physical, psychological, mental, and spiritual aspects of the energy field. These dysfunctions can be sensed by the practitioner of Healing Touch as areas of energy blockage or deficiency experienced as coolness or absence of vibration. Or there may be a congestion of energy, a bulge of heat, experienced as excess on assessment. The blockage may affect only the outer dimensions of the field signifying spiritual disconnectedness, or it may reach into the mental dimension in the form of faulty thought patterns. In the emotional dimension, constrictions in the chakra field imply negative attitudes and feelings that may become part of a personality pattern or mood disorder over time. Finally, blockage may affect the physical body in the form of symptoms of dis-

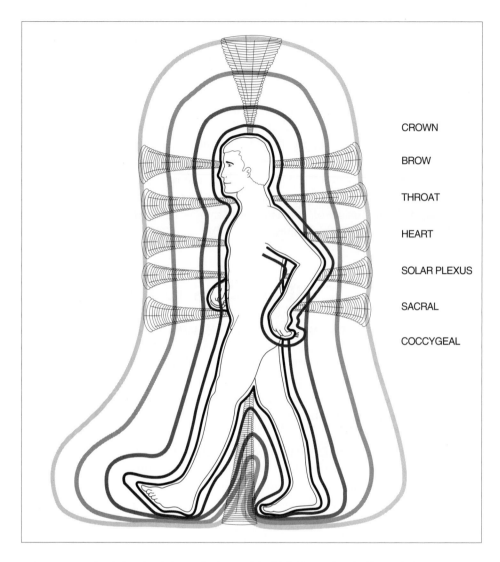

CROWN

BROW

THROAT

HEART

SOLAR PLEXUS

SACRAL

COCCYGEAL

**FIGURE 6.1** The chakras in relation to the layers of the biofield. (Reprinted with permission from Janet L. Mentgen, Program Administrator, Healing Touch)

ease. Table 6.3 shows the major dysfunctions in each related layer of the field as a simple guide for the healing practitioner.

Another useful assessment tool is to sense the condition of each chakra individually. Alice Bailey (1978), describes five major conditions of the chakras in her somewhat metaphorical style:

1. CLOSED, still and shut, yet with signs of life, silent and full of deep inertia.

| TABLE 6.2 | Optimum Function of Each Chakra and Related Field | | | |
|---|---|---|---|---|
| **Chakra** | **Physical** | **Emotional** | **Mental** | **Spiritual** |
| Coccygeal or Root | Vital life energy flow<br><br>Ability to respond to stressors | Realistic and appropriate trust<br><br>Responds with appropriate emotions to life events<br><br>Full enjoyment of being alive | "I am secure."<br><br>"I belong on the earth."<br><br>"I deserve to enjoy my life fully." | The universe is friendly. |
| Sacral | Fluid assimilation, elimination, and balance<br><br>Sexual enjoyment | Positive self-image<br><br>Able to sort out relationships and establish close bonds | Discrimination of positive and negative<br><br>"I choose; I select."<br><br>Able to release unwanted feelings | Everything is open to choice.<br><br>Cocreation |
| Solar Plexus | Good digestion and utilization of nutrients<br><br>Muscles in harmony<br><br>"Bounce" in walk | Balance of masculine and feminine aspects of personality<br><br>Flexibility<br><br>Sense of direction<br><br>Ability to set goals and complete activity | "I am in charge of my life."<br><br>"My energy is steady to accomplish my goals." | Work with laws of attraction |

| TABLE 6.2 | Optimum Function of Each Chakra and Related Field (continued) | | | |
| --- | --- | --- | --- | --- |
| **Chakra** | **Physical** | **Emotional** | **Mental** | **Spiritual** |
| Heart | Sense of well-being<br><br>Lightness, radiance in appearance<br><br>Good posture | Forgives easily<br><br>Able to send and receive love<br><br>Feeling of satisfaction | "I am lovable and capable."<br><br>"I forgive easily." | Awareness of the reality of the soul<br><br>Radiant love |
| Throat | Full, rich sound in voice<br><br>Creativity | Enjoys expressing self<br><br>Willing to take risks<br><br>Effective communi-cation | Values own and others' ideas<br><br>Enjoys sharing and teaching | Expresses soul's nature and purpose |
| Brow | Open, alert appearance<br><br>Perception of details, beauty | Compassion for others<br><br>Insight<br><br>Sensitivity<br><br>Sense of humor | Evaluates without judging<br><br>"I see clearly."<br><br>Plans ahead | The universe makes sense. |
| Crown | All energy centers open and flowing<br><br>Body systems in harmony | Kinship with others<br><br>Concern for all of human kind<br><br>Joy and deep feelings | "I am one with the one."<br><br>Higher sense perception | Mystical experiences<br><br>Unitive glimpses merging with divine will |

| TABLE 6.3 | Dysfunctions in Each Chakra and Related Field | | | |
|---|---|---|---|---|
| Chakra | Physical | Emotional | Mental | Spiritual |
| Coccygeal or Root | Fatigue<br><br>Lack of body awareness<br><br>Ailments of low back, hips, legs, perineum | Greed<br><br>Apathy<br><br>Lack of energy, intensity, vitality<br><br>Fear | Poor concentration<br><br>Confusion<br><br>Lack of motivation<br><br>Passivity | Lack of purpose, meaning, or direction in life. |
| Sacral | Fluid imbalance<br><br>Edema<br><br>Chemical dependency<br><br>Sexual disorders | Gullibility<br><br>Hanging on<br><br>Defensiveness<br><br>Sexual disorders<br><br>Codependency | Difficulty differentiating positive and negative<br><br>Poor relationship skills<br><br>Resentments | Victim consciousness<br><br>Belief in fate<br><br>Predetermination |
| Solar Plexus | Tension in muscles<br><br>Addictions<br><br>Stress disorders<br><br>Digestive problems | Competitive<br><br>Driven<br><br>Compulsive<br><br>Perfectionistic<br><br>Domineering | Controlling<br><br>Power-hungry<br><br>Unable to trust others<br><br>"I'm the only one who can do it right." | Aloneness<br><br>No trust in Higher Power |
| Heart | Chest pain<br><br>Stooped posture to protect heart<br><br>Cardiovascular disease<br><br>Immune disorders | Guilt<br><br>Holding grudges<br><br>Sorrow<br><br>Loneliness<br><br>Vengefulness | "Others should make me happy."<br><br>"No one can love me enough." | Karmic indebtedness<br><br>Trapped — no way out<br><br>Have to earn love |

| TABLE 6.3 | Dysfunctions in Each Chakra and Related Field (continued) | | | |

| Chakra | Physical | Emotional | Mental | Spiritual |
|---|---|---|---|---|
| Throat | "Pinched" voice tone<br><br>Hoarseness<br><br>Throat problems | Unexpressive<br><br>Poor self-esteem<br><br>Closed, dull<br><br>Unwilling to risk | "If I express myself, something terrible will happen."<br><br>"Others are better than me." | "Universe is unfriendly and unsafe." |
| Brow | Visual, sensory problems<br><br>Sinus and headache problems<br><br>Difficulty with details | Poor insight<br><br>Difficulty putting self in others' place | Rationalistic<br><br>Concrete thinking<br><br>Literal<br><br>Critical and judgmental | God is judgment<br><br>There is a great critic out there |
| Crown | Minimal dysfunction as we are always connnected to the Universal Energy Field. Some dysfunctions observed: | | | |
| | Poor assimilation from UEF<br><br>Lack of vitality | Constricting emotions<br><br>Feeling "lost" | Limited thinking<br><br>"I don't deserve the best." | Disconnected<br><br>View of God as too small and impersonal |

2. OPENING, unsealed, and faintly tinged with color; the life pulsates.
3. QUICKENED, alive, alert in two directions; the two small doors are open wide.
4. RADIANT and reaching forth with vibrant note to all related centers.
5. BLENDED they are and each with each works rhythmically. The vital force flows through from all the planes. (p. 81)

These poetic descriptions from a great teacher give us some idea of the excitement of determining the state of each center. As we identify the state of the chakra — closed, opening, quickened, radiant, or blended — we can relate each center to its impact in the energy field. Further assessment of the field as a whole gives us an energy-based and intuitive perception of what is occurring with the client.

# CHAKRA MEDITATION

Progressing upward starting from the base of the spine:

**Chakra 1**
> My mind is firm
> And steadfast like a rock.
> I am secure, and safe
> Able to withstand all shock.

**Chakra 2**
> My body energy flows at my command,
> Emotions balanced, Mastery is in my hand.

**Chakra 3**
> I rise to meet obstacles —
> My path is clear.
> I trust my guidance
> Control is here.

**Chakra 4**
> What can hold, constrict, or encumber me?
> Nothing of this world: I am free. I am free!

**Chakra 5**
> Awake! My sleeping powers within, Arise!
> Like the wind in the trees, God's power within me lies.

**Chakra 6**
> My soul flows
> On waves of cosmic light.
> My insight expands,
> Intuition is right.

**Chakra 7**
> My silence is an expanding wave
> Of cosmic light —
> Above, below, without, within,
> To the left and to the right —
> Everywhere
> The universe lives within my peace.

# Chakra Exercise

This is an example of the many ways you can experience your own chakra awareness and sense movement in your own energy body.

1. Allow yourself to center and feel grounded to the earth. Begin by spreading your hands on your thighs, bending your knees, and sensing the connection to the earth through the outflow of *Qi* from your hands and feet.

2. Sense the inflow of *Qi* from the Universal Energy Field into your heart center and your hands, which may be held facing each other over the heart center as you focus with a sense of gratitude and thanksgiving. Remember that there are strong energy vortices in the palms of the hands and soles of the feet.

3. Bring the *Qi* from the heart center to the root chakra area at the base of the spine, while affirming your joy of being alive in the physical body. If desired, add a vigorous spin as you would if you were moving a "hula hoop."

4. Now, allow *Qi* to flow from your hands to the sacral center, front and back. Affirm your ability to select and choose the nutrients, people, and situations that are right for you. Continue rotating while focusing on the sacral area.

5. Bring your awareness and your hands to the solar plexus with its strengths for taking charge and communicating effectively. Add a slight rotation while feeling your own power.

6. Let *Qi* now flow freely from your hands to the heart center, enjoying a sense of acceptance and forgiveness. Imagine reaching out to your loved ones and then bringing in their caring with large arm movements.

7. Bring the hands over the throat center, front and back, while sensing support from the Universal Energy Field for your creativity. Allow your voice to make a sound, finding the tone that is most pleasing to you. Try all five vowels with this tone, play with sound.

8. Allow the hands to rest above the brow chakra, both front and back, affirming your ability to develop higher sense perception and to see with insight and compassion.

9. Bring the hands to the crown while feeling the inflow of *Qi* from the Universal. Sense the connection with infinite peace, love, and wisdom for your unique life, and its meaning and purpose.

# SUMMARY

As we become more at ease in determining chakra and energy field interactions, we begin to notice certain patterns within each individual, almost like a psychic signature. In the next chapter we will explore the implications of these patterns for the work of understanding the client's needs. The selection of actual healing techniques can be made effectively when the healer has a good knowledge and skill base in assessing and understanding the functions of the chakras and biofield. We will explore specific applications of this knowledge in the third section of the book, which provides a variety of techniques for healing.

# REFERENCES

Bailey, A. (1978). *Esoteric healing*. New York: Lucis Publishing Co.

Besant, A., & Leadbeater, C. W. (1925). *Thought forms*. Wheaton, IL: Theosophical Publishing House.

Brennan, B. (1987). *Hands of light*. New York: Bantam Books.

Bruyere, R. (1989). *Wheels of light*. Arcadia, CA: Bon Productions.

Eden, D. (1998). *Energy medicine*. New York: Tarcher/Putnam, 133–171.

Judith, A. (1996). *Eastern body, western mind*. Berkeley, CA: Celestial Arts.

Liberman, J. (1991). *Light: Medicine of the future*. Santa Fe, NM: Bear & Co.

Motoyama, H. (1995). *Theories of the chakras*. Wheaton, IL: Theosophical Publishing House.

Motoyama, H. (1999). *Comparisons of diagnostic methods in western and eastern medicine*. Tokyo, Japan: Human Science Press.

Rama, S., Ballentine, R., & Ajaya, S. (1981). *Yoga and psychotherapy* (p. 217). Honesdale, PA: Himalayan International Institute.

Reilly, H. J., & Brod, R. (1975). *The Edgar Cayce handbook for health*. New York: Macmillan Publishing.

Sherwood, K. (1996). *Chakra theory for personal growth and healing*. St. Paul, MN: Llewellyn.

Slater, V. (2000). Energetic Healing. In Dossey, B. et al. (Eds.), *Holistic nursing*. Gaithersburg, MD: Aspen Publishers, 132–141.

Tamarkin, L., Baird, C., & Almeida, O. F. (1985). Melantonin: A coordinating signal for mammalian reproduction. *Science, 227*.

Tansley, D. V. (1985). *Subtle body*. New York: Thames and Hudson.

# CHAPTER 7

# Assessing and Identifying Patterns in the Biofield and Chakras

*"The interweaving of the three fields of the personal self, together with their vehicle, the physical body, gives us a picture of human life which can be compared to a moving four-dimensional tapestry, whose warp and woof are composed of threads of differing qualities and textures and whose patterns shift and change as they cut across the path of time. The key to understanding the complexity of this process of interaction lies in its dynamism, for life is always characterized by growth and change."*

—Karagulla & Kunz, 1989

## INTRODUCTION

The metaphor of the interweaving energy dimensions implies that there are distinctive patterns unique to the consciousness of each individual. As the healer begins to assess the biofield and each chakra, she can perceive an image while doing a hand scan that gives a profile of the individual's energy field. This feedback from the field allows the healer to quickly identify characteristics related to the individual. After assessment is complete, one can make some inferences from the energy pattern to predominant psychological and physical issues in the client.

The practitioner uses the knowledge gained from understanding the functions of the chakras and their condition to make a holistic, integrative assessment. The healer's own preparation for this work is self-awareness through centering and meditation, which we will discuss more thoroughly in later parts of this book.

## IDENTIFYING PATTERNS IN THE BIOFIELD

The word *intuition* is derived from the Latin *intueri*, which means to consider or look within. True intuition is the function of a person who has developed higher levels of consciousness through daily attention to meditative practice. As intellectual knowledge of the energy system and wisdom of the higher sense perception combine, the healer can become highly skilled in identifying needs of the client.

In this chapter we will explore some of the energetic patterns that can readily be perceived with experience and training. This discussion is naturally not intended to label any particular individual, as we see all persons as evolving, dynamic entities. The emphasis here is on understanding information received from the sample energy fields described and seeing how assessment and visual documentation give direction to healing interventions.

## Effect of Blocked Chakras

As we discussed in the previous chapter, the chakras are the receptive points that allow the inflow and outflow of energy from the Universal Energy Field. If this receptor is blocked for any reason the client may be receiving an inadequate supply of supportive life force and may develop a depletion of $Qi$ in the physical or emotional dimensions that are associated with the chakra's functioning. Over time, a compensation for this depletion may develop in the form of an overabundance, or excess of $Qi$, in another chakra. Like the genetic code that is inherent in every cell through the RNA and DNA molecules, the imprint of one or more closed, blocked chakras creates a pattern throughout the entire vibrational matrix. By way of analogy, consider how a motif, or basic theme, in music is repeated and integrated throughout an entire composition. We can also speak of certain basic patterns in the collective human psyche, called archetypes by Jung, that are repeated and developed within each individual's lifetime. Embedded constrictions of the energy field can be carried by the client for many years unless there is intentional correction or repatterning.

## Making an Energy-Oriented Assessment

The purpose of assessment in Healing Touch practice is to define the areas of imbalance in the biofield and chakras that help direct the healer's plan of care. In the art and science of nursing, the nursing diagnosis is the foundation for planning, intervention, and evaluation. Nursing diagnosis is prescriptive for planning nursing interventions, in contrast to a medical diagnosis which determines the medical treatment plan. HT practitioners make an assessment of $Qi$ patterns, noting areas of depletion or of excess, patterns of constricted, stagnated energy, or smooth-flowing areas. This assessment becomes the basis for implementing HT interventions.

"Energy field disturbance" has been an accepted nursing diagnosis since 1995 (NANDA, 1995–1996) and is well-documented in nursing literature. It lends a purposeful cornerstone to Healing Touch practice as well. Day to day charting of a client's progress can be facilitated by specific descriptions of energetic disturbances described in this chapter. The interventions and techniques of Healing Touch, from the generic to the specific, are based on the energetic assessment and permit the healer to evaluate changes in the client's patterning.

# ASSESSING THE BIOFIELD AND CHAKRAS

Learning to sense a client's energy field requires clarity, centering, development of our intuitive talents, and much practice. We are speaking here of the sensing of subtle vibrations that have just recently been found to be measurable by sensitive scientific technology. There will be no claps of thunder or neon lights; each therapist learns to define a way of sensing energy that is relevant to her cognitive thinking style.

All of the perceptive senses can come into play as the healer develops ways of describing fine and subtle energies. However, the caregiver may initially need to rely on her predominant perceptual system. We begin new learning from our point of comfort and our favorite way of talking about experience (Bandler & Grinder, 1985). Thus, a predominantly visual person would begin to "see," looking for the nuances and shadings around the client's physical body. Some highly skilled visual healers learn to see the colors of the aura, differentiating areas of darkness or light in relation to each chakra. On the other hand, an auditory individual might begin to sense areas of harmony and disharmony by picking up sounds in the energy field. Most healers are highly kinesthetic and are very comfortable with sensory perception through the hands. Some become very adept at distinguishing areas of fullness around an open chakra and areas of absence of this fullness suggesting a closed or obstructed chakra.

To use another description, the healer may sense warmth or a tingling vibration in a radiant, open center and coolness and less tingling in a closed center. Whatever mode of accessing sensory data is initially used, the healer learns to add the other perceptual systems to get a wide range of feedback from the client. Thus, the vibrational patterns of the energy field are accessible through our own learning of higher sense perception. Practice, and plenty of it, with healthy persons and comparisons with someone who is ill, is the best teacher.

Whatever means of assessment are used, the hands of the healer are the tools. The compassion of the healer is the perceiver. The mind of the healer is the interpreter. And the spirit or soul of the healer is the guide.

## Documentation

A method or system of noting each observation is important. Symbols for the condition of each chakra can be used, such as a period for a chakra that is completely closed and circles of varying sizes to describe the degree of opening and intensity of the spin of the chakra, which is usually clockwise in a healthy chakra. It is also useful to make a visual representation or profile of the entire energy system. This assists us in recognizing significant patterns that relate to physical and emotional issues.

# PHYSICAL PROBLEMS AS PATTERNS IN THE BIOFIELD

## Immune System Deficiency

One dramatic illness that completely depletes the immune system is AIDS, Acquired Immunodeficiency Syndrome. The AIDS epidemic has mandated that we understand the immune system and its dysfunctions more fully. Here, a complex and often mutating retrovirus attacks the body's major immune cells, such as the T-4, and destroys them, leaving the victim subject to a vast array of opportunistic infections. In fact, AIDS sufferers do not die from the action of the virus but from the effects of some otherwise innocuous organism, such as the *Pneumocystis carinii,* that takes over when the body's usual defenses are missing.

Other physical illnesses also cause depletion or a shutting down of the immune system with an impact on the energy field. Chronic infections with long-term side effects or overexposure to environmental pollution override the defenders of the body. Cancer, the unchecked growth of abnormal cells, is another disease that drains and deprives the body of its immune resources.

Immune system deficiency has devastating effects on the energy field and the vitality of the individual. This deficiency in the field can be sensed by the Healing Touch therapist as an emptiness, a flatness, or lack of "bounce," especially in the lower centers. The higher centers—throat, brow, and crown—may often be overactive to compensate for the lack of vitality in the lower centers. We sometimes call this predominance of the mental centers "running on mental energy," which is a very apt description of what happens energetically.

Figure 7.1 suggests a way of mapping an immune deficiency pattern that was sensed by the hands of the healer in the field of an AIDS patient. The lack of energy can often be sensed in the emotional and causal fields as well. Knowing the basic pattern and its effect can guide the therapist to implement ways of bringing vitality back through hands-on techniques like the Full Body Connection, which we will describe in the next section.

## Autoimmune Diseases

A wide variety of physical dysfunctions, called autoimmune diseases, result from an excessive immune response. In this instance, the systemic immune response is excessive and certain cells actually begin to attack the body. Examples of autoimmune diseases are lupus erythematosus, rheumatoid arthritis, some demyelinizing syndromes, and severe allergic reactions leading to asthma attacks.

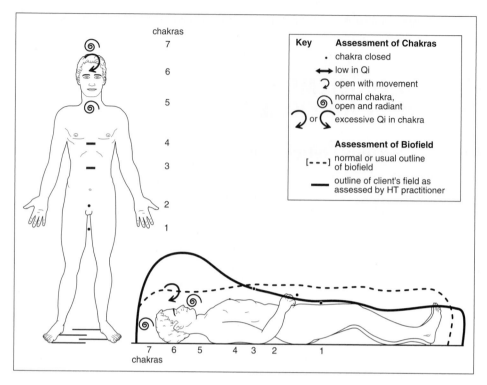

**FIGURE 7.1**  Energetic pattern of the immune system dysfunction

Chronic Fatigue Syndrome is currently understood as an autoimmune disease in which the body responds to viral and environmental stresses by being "on" all the time, thus depleting the endocrine glands, the thyroid and adrenals particularly, and exhausting the client's physical resources (NANDA, 1994).

In the case of autoimmune disease, the therapist may hear the client describe symptoms of fatigue, achiness, and vague distress with a complementary lack of vitality in the entire energy field. A client with this problem will take on energy rapidly with healing interventions, resulting in a sense of well-being and relief. However, this may only last a few minutes as the individual is unable to store the energy. It is helpful in autoimmune diseases to teach a family member or signifi-cant other how to facilitate maintaining energy balance. Eventually, through repeated working with the biofield, the client learns to maintain a steady flow of supportive and life-sustaining vitality. Over time this may permit a repatterning of the field toward more balance and wholeness.

## Cardiovascular Problems

As heart disease is the leading cause of sudden, unexpected deaths in the United States, energy field assessment is valuable in detecting early warning signals. In heart disease, the imprint of a chakra's diminished functioning can be noted in the emotional and mental dimensions of the field. This change in energy levels can be sensed before physical symptoms, like angina or left quadrant pain, appear prior to a full-blown heart attack. As a matter of fact, many medical practitioners are beginning to note early warning signs in the emotional dimension by obtaining a full history of the client's lifestyle pattern.

***The Type A Personality***    The Type A personality (Friedman & Rosenmann, 1974) is characteristic of an individual who learns to protect an emotionally wounded heart by overcompensating in other areas of life. Typically, this person feels driven to achieve, pushing herself and others unmercifully. This person may be a leader in her company who is domineering and compulsive, or a tyrant in her family. As others move away, she may push harder, which only drives others to further avoidance. The real need—to be loved and accepted unconditionally—is unmet and the person may feel embittered and alone.

From an energetic point of view, the Type A personality presents an excess of *Qi* in the solar plexus chakra. This can also be apparent in the biofield, and the heart chakra may be weakened or closed. Often, the lower centers dealing with trust levels, survival issues, and sexual expression are depleted or shut down whereas the mental processes, especially the brow center, predominate as if to compensate for the missing pieces.

Figure 7.2 shows the profile of a counseling client who fit this personality pattern. Because he was in the early stages of its onset, coming in for marital problems initially, much could be done to assist him in making lifestyle changes. By working through early childhood and career issues, he was able to reactivate the full function of the blocked centers and to achieve emotional harmony in his life. A good physical examination was also imperative to check for possible physical damage, such as hypertension or circulatory disorders, and to begin his program of health awareness.

We begin to see, then, how assessment of a pattern can give the clues to needed lifestyle changes in the physical, emotional, and mental aspects toward balance of energy. This repatterning of the entire field appears to result in increasing levels of wellness and health.

# High Stress Patterns

High levels of stress and emotional pressure are so prevalent that it is almost redundant to remind clients that stress may be affecting their sense of vitality and the biofield as a whole. It is usually easy to detect the signature of stress in the energy field if there is an absence of other physical symptoms. Constriction or closing of the root chakra is an obvious sign. The adrenals, which are programmed to respond to aversive stimuli, become overactive as pressure and the feeling of being threatened accumulate. When the adrenals have had too much stimulation, the body takes over with compensatory mechanisms, such as high

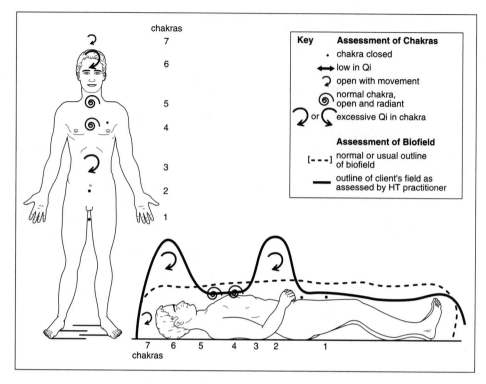

**FIGURE 7.2** Energy pattern of Type A personality (often called the "successful person" in our culture)

blood pressure, that become generalized and systemic (Selye, 1978; Stuart-Shortwells-Federman, 2000, pp. 379–382).

In figure 7.3 we see the profile of a young woman whose boss constantly harassed her. Her wish to do well kept her in this untenable position until she developed panic attacks and nightmares, which led her to seek counseling. The root chakra was completely blocked, and she expressed fear that she might not live long; her very survival was being threatened by the work situation. She attempted to compensate by trying harder, which caused an overexertion of the solar plexus, and by trying to be unconditionally loving, which taxed the heart center.

Fortunately, the emotional needs drove her to seek appropriate help before the problems led to physical disease. Many individuals can be helped by learning to relax, activating autogenic responses, and practicing biofeedback (Green & Green, 1977; Anselmo & Kolkmeier, 2000, pp. 519–523). Changes in lifestyle patterns can further help the client to relieve distress and, ultimately, to bring the energy field to higher balance.

Medical practitioners usually see persons with more advanced symptomatology—high blood pressure, headaches, glaucoma, adrenal or kidney dysfunctions. From an energetic point of view, we can see why just treating the condition with

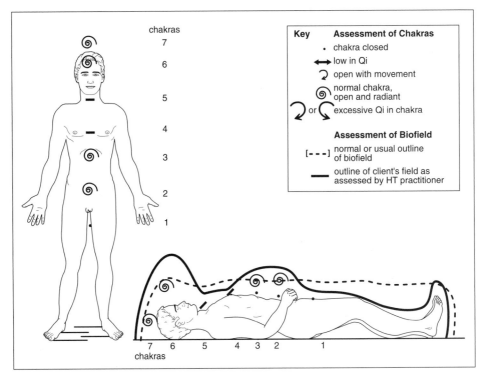

**FIGURE 7.3** Energy pattern related to high stress

medication would be insufficient. Beyond lifestyle changes and health education, the individual must find ways to increase the inner sense of security and of safety, to open the root center, and to allow a full flow of *Qi* to all the higher centers.

# EMOTIONAL ISSUES IN THE BIOFIELD

## Grief and Depression

Although grief and depression are predominantly emotional symptoms, they also have physical concomitants that most people recognize. Grief is a natural, emotional response to the loss of a loved one. As such it is not an abnormal state, although many individuals are surprised at the wide variety of strange thoughts, emotions, and physical symptoms that can occur. A healthy expression of grief diminishes over time and the individual can begin to reconnect with family and friends in new ways. An unhealthy grief reaction is one that persists over time (often well over several years), does not diminish in intensity, is denied, or is incapacitating to the individual.

Grief has a distinctive energetic pattern in which the lower centers are diminished or blocked for a period of time with a concomitant loss of enjoyment of life and lowering of libido. Figure 7.4 shows the energy field profile of a client who was newly widowed with two young children in her charge. Needless to say, her entire world was upside down and shattered. She needed to literally rebuild her life in a new way. We can note the lowered energy levels in the entire field and a general harmony of the upper chakras, as there had not been time to develop adaptations or overcompensations.

When we see a similar pattern in a person who has not experienced a significant loss recently, we may think of looking for repressed grief. Often, the denial of mourning means that the individual never shed all the tears that needed to be released. The sadness is held as a constriction or block in the biofield. The person may feel too overwhelmed to bring the sadness to awareness and develops major constrictions as time goes on. Depression is often a suppressed form of grief, a generalized adaptation, in which the individual is sad and functioning at half-strength most of the time.

## Codependency and Childhood Abuse

Much has been written recently about personality patterns of individuals who grew up in dysfunctional families and later moved into distorted relationships in

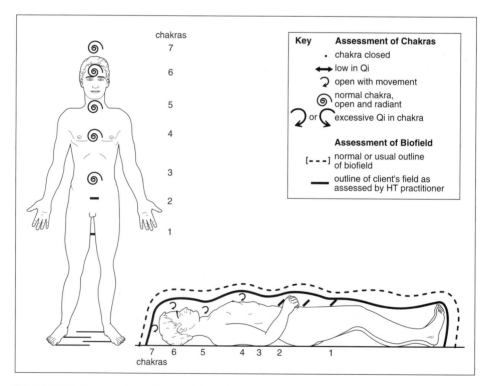

**FIGURE 7.4** Energy pattern of acute grief reaction

adulthood (Beattie, 1987; Black, 1982). It is not surprising, then, that these patterns can be sensed in the biofield. The heart and sexual centers are usually wide open or overfilled with *Qi* indicating the indiscriminate giving of love and affection even to unworthy parents or partners. The intuitive center, the brow chakra, is diminished or blocked so that the codependent cannot see with insight into others' motivations or realities.

Represented in figure 7.5 is the energetic description of a client who was compulsively attracted to abusive men. Until evaluation of the field was done, she was not consciously aware of the abuse that occurred in early childhood. The energy pattern showed tremendous blocks in the pelvic area; holding in of the power center, the solar plexus; and signs of long-term imbalance in that every dimension of the field was affected. When this was brought to her attention in a safe and supportive environment, she began to recall, in short flashes, scenes of very early abuse that she could not comprehend or verbalize.

The lifetime impact of childhood abuse can be seen in the extreme distortions of the energy field. We are just beginning to comprehend the devastating effects of abuse that leave behind a legacy of distorted thinking and emotional patterns (Whitfield, 1987). We know it can take years to counteract these distortions through psychotherapy. From an energy-based point of view, we can assist the client in releasing old memories, which are literally blocks in the energy field, so

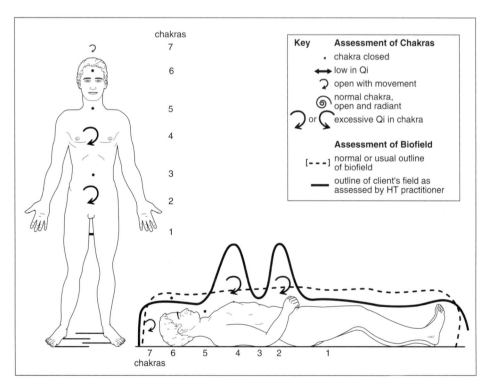

**FIGURE 7.5** Energy pattern associated with codependency and childhood abuse

that new thinking and feeling patterns can emerge. We will further explore the integration of psychotherapy and energy concepts in chapter 15.

## Being Strong

In our culture denying feelings and being strong are highly valued. This thinking is further enhanced in the educational process of many health care professionals who are taught to be objective and impersonal at all times. Treating a patient as a diagnosis or an object to be moved from one technology to another preserves this kind of distancing. Unfortunately, the very qualities of human warmth and caring that could most help the patient are denied with this philosophy. Although holding in one's feelings may not cause active distress, it definitely blocks the flow of *Qi* in the chakras and the field, creating a kind of invisible barrier that prevents the intuitive, creative potential and the capacity to enjoy life fully to emerge.

Many persons who have lived with such barriers in their biofields experience vague symptoms of dissatisfaction. These may become more apparent in midlife when one begins asking, "Is this all there is?" Thus, what is often termed *midlife crisis* is another time to take stock of our human energies and to explore ways of opening safely to wider awareness, our sense of true purpose, and meaning in life.

## SUMMARY

We begin to note that energetic assessment is a valuable complement to traditional medical and psychological care. It is not enough simply to medicate or give talk-therapy. Use of purposeful energetic techniques to release blockages can speed the healing process for the client. This has rich implications for working with medical practitioners, body-oriented therapists, and psychotherapists. With a combination of appropriate energetic interventions and traditional practices, the client can move more quickly and effectively into desired personal change and prevent physical breakdown.

## REFERENCES

Anselmo, J. & Kolkmeier, L. G. (2000). In Dossey, B. et al. (Eds.) *Holistic nursing*, Gaithersburg, MD: Aspen Publishers.

Bandler, R., & Grinder, J. (1995). *Using your brain for a change*. Moab, UT: Real People Press.

Beattie, M. (1987). *Codependent no more*. New York: Harper and Row.

Benson, H. (1997). *Timeless healing*. New York: Fireside.

Black, C. (1982). *It will never happen to me!* Denver: M.A.C. Printing and Publications Division.

Friedman, M., & Rosenmann, R. H. (1974). *Type A behavior and your heart.* Greenwich, CT: Fawcett Publishing.

Green, E., & Green, A. (1977). *Beyond biofeedback.* New York: Delta Books.

Karagulla, S., & Kunz, D. (1989). *The chakras and the human energy fields.* Wheaton, IL: Theosophical Publishing House. p. 27.

North American Nursing Diagnosis Association (NANDA), *NANDA nursing diagnoses: Definitions and classification, 1995–1996.* Philadelphia, PA: NANDA Publications.

Selye, H. (1978). *The stress of life.* New York: American Library.

Stuart-Shor, E. M. & Wells-Federman, C. L. (2000). In Dossey, B. et al. (Eds.), *Holistic nursing.* Gaithersburg, MD: Aspen Publishers.

Whitfield, C. L. (1987). *Healing the child within.* Deerfield Beach, FL: Health Communications, Inc.

-----, (1994). A guide to CFIDS (chronic immune deficiency syndrome), *CFIDS Chronicle*, Winter, 57–58.

# Basic Applications for Healing Interventions

*"Centering is the healer's most essential resource—the focus of intention and goodwill on behalf of the client."*

—Dorothea Hover-Kramer

## INTRODUCTION

There are unlimited applications in healing practice of the chakra and biofield concepts we have discussed. Before moving into the specific Healing Touch interventions given in section III, we will look in this chapter at the most basic interventions for healing. These have been known throughout human history whenever there was genuine desire to help another person, and have been handed down through oral and written traditions, becoming more refined and complex as they addressed more specific human needs.

All healing approaches involve some form of inner *focusing*, or centering, to access the practitioner's positive intent. In addition, usually some means of *assessment* of the client's energy pattern is used to determine areas of blockage or disruption of the flow of *Qi*. Based on the assessment, the practitioner then proceeds with *clearing* or *smoothing* of the biofield to relieve a blocked or congested area and with *modulation* of energy on or over the affected area. We will explore these basic concepts along with learning exercises that allow you to practice developing your sensitivity before moving into the specific steps of the many Healing Touch interventions. But, before we go further, we wish to acknowledge the pioneering efforts of the Therapeutic Touch community in setting the accessible, excellent groundwork for the many energy-linked healing modalities.

## THERAPEUTIC TOUCH

In 1970, nursing professor Dr. Dolores Krieger began introducing basic concepts of energy healing to her nursing students at New York University. She worked with her partner, Dora Kunz, a natural intuitive healer who had assisted many physicians before the days of noninvasive medical imaging, to establish

Therapeutic Touch as, what they called, "a contemporary interpretation of several ancient healing practices. These practices consist of learned skills for consciously directing or sensitively modulating human energies" (Krieger, 1993, p. 11).

Because of the innovative nature of the program thirty years ago when energy concepts were relatively unknown, there were many skeptics. Dr. Krieger's students called themselves "Krieger's Krazies" as a way of showing their special camaraderie while their colleagues puzzled over these methods. Over time, however, the truth of the work has stood firm, and the effects have been experienced by hundreds of thousands of patients in reducing pain and anxiety, in promoting relaxation, and in enhancing the body's natural restorative processes. In the health care field, Therapeutic Touch, as developed by Krieger and Kunz, is the best-known and foremost energetic approach to healing. It is taught in over 80 major universities and colleges in the United States and is recognized in over 60 other countries. It has become the support and research base for the many new energetic modalities that include the practice of Healing Touch.

The most basic intervention of Therapeutic Touch, a nine-step procedure with four dynamic, interactive phases, is used to assist clients to repattern their energies toward enhanced balance (Nurse Healers—Professional Associates, Inc., 2000). Usually, 15 to 20 minutes is considered ample time for a treatment and the practitioner adjusts the intervention to the needs of the client. In general, neonates, children, pregnant women, persons with psychiatric disorders, the elderly, and the acutely ill are more sensitive and therefore may need such modifications as briefer time periods or less emphatic movements on the part of the practitioner.

The organization that represents and supports Therapeutic Touch practitioners is the Nurse Healers—Professional Associates International, Inc. (See Appendix B for more contact information). The organization has developed its *Policy and Procedure Manual* to define its practitioners as those who have successfully completed basic levels of training and mentorship on the theory and practice of Therapeutic Touch, and currently has a teacher cooperative, guidelines of the development of practitioners and teachers, and criteria for endorsing its programs (as reported in Nurse Healers, 2000, p. 2).

Because Therapeutic Touch and Healing Touch have similar names and have related roots in energy–based healing concepts, there is often confusion about the two programs. Simply stated, Therapeutic Touch is the original energy healing philosophy developed by Krieger and Kunz over thirty years ago that has spawned many emerging programs. Healing Touch is a younger first cousin developed by Janet Mentgen and her many associates. It began eleven years ago and is a compilation of the work of many healers, including Brugh Joy, Rosalyn Bruyere, and Barbara Brennan, as well as the intuitive healing methods that have emerged spontaneously from its many practitioners. As noted in the first chapter, Healing Touch is also a program of sequenced learning activities leading to certification through its international association (described in Appendix B).

The basic processes that we will identify in this chapter are similar to some of many Therapeutic Touch interventions, but are not intended to preempt the extensive learning and insight skills that are required to become a Therapeutic Touch practitioner and to learn its integrative methods. Each program has its unique aspects and founding orientation. Healing work, as we have noted in the history chapter, is a universal concept that lies in the public domain. We begin here with basic tools that allow you to understand how we integrate energy theory with healing practices. These skills form the basic framework for the specific, and more original Healing Touch techniques given in the next section.

# BASIC PROCESSES

The exercises in this chapter give you an opportunity to learn about focusing/centering, assessing the biofield, smoothing or clearing, modulating energy, and bringing about closure. In subsequent chapters, you will see ways you can use each of these processes individually or integrate them into a longer healing session in conjunction with many other techniques.

## Sensing Energy

Sensing your own biofield is a good way to begin learning about energy. The steps described in the following exercise give you a way to practice increasing your sensitivity and to learn from your own experience. With practice, it can teach you much about your own energy field and enhance your sensitivity to energy. The exercise also requires focusing your attention by working with the breath, paying attention to the body, and refocusing whenever your attention wanders. Needless to say, this is not easy the first time, but it becomes much more natural with repetition and practice.

Essentially, you are learning how to bring the restless, sometimes wandering mind into calmer, more focused attention. We call this *centering*, and it is the basic tool for all energetic interventions whether for self-care or to assist others.

EXERCISE

## SENSING ENERGY

1. Begin by taking several deep breaths, being careful to exhale completely, as if releasing air from a balloon. Blow out gently as if you were blowing out a candle. Sense the release of tension as you exhale, and connect with the joy of nature as you inhale.

2. Image bringing golden sunlight into your lungs as you inhale and releasing any darkness or heaviness as you exhale. Let the golden

*(continues)*

*(continued)*

light flow to your heart, and, with the blood's circulation, image the flow of the light to each part of your body. Note anywhere there is discomfort or a constriction in your body.

3.  See the golden light flowing from the center of your chest to the shoulders, the arms, and the hands. Let the hands fill with the unlimited flow of this golden light and the quality of warmth and caring.

4.  Maintaining your relaxed state, bring the palms of the hands opposite each other. Sense the fullness or warmth between them. Note how far you can separate the hands and still feel this fullness or warmth. Note how close together you can bring the hands without touching. Is there a difference? Explore the sensation, letting go of any goal or need to "do it right."

5.  Continuing your work with gentle breaths to refocus whenever your attention wanders, bring your awareness into the right index finger. Let the finger point at the left palm and draw a pattern at a distance of 1–3 inches as seen in figure 8.1. Note how this feels.

6.  Bring your full attention into the left index finger and send your awareness into the right palm drawing another pattern. How does this feel? Is one hand more sensitive to sending or receiving than the other?

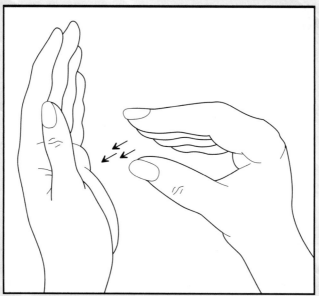

**FIGURE 8.1** Sensing energy by directing index finger into opposite palm.

*(continues)*

*(continued)*

7. Gently bring your focus back to the palms of both hands. Let them play back and forth as you observe your experience. Simply let yourself enjoy the awareness and discovery from your own energies.

8. Bring the energized hands to rest on any part of the body that felt uncomfortable earlier. Continue to draw the golden light from the limitless universe into your body with the breath and your caring attention.

9. Gently release your focus and come back to the present making a note of what you have learned.

## Centering

Practitioners of energy-oriented modalities find that centering, working with inner awareness, is the most vital part of their work. If we are centered, we can move with confidence and a full, flowing, protective energy field into difficult situations. If we are off-center and discombobulated, we stumble around, becoming more and more frazzled with less and less to give. Energetically speaking, centering brings us into harmony with the Universal Energy Flow. Even without specific knowledge of energies, others can sense the difference when we are in a state of balance.

The exercise for centering is specifically designed to help you learn to develop your inner focus and later learn to do it quickly in clinical settings. With practice, this kind of daily centering gives you a delightful way to begin or end the day or to calm yourself during a break in the work schedule. It is a good idea to practice every day for 15 minutes until it becomes a natural part of your daily routine, like brushing your teeth. More rapid centering, at a patient's beside for instance, is possible after the longer method becomes automatic. With practice, just taking an intentional breath and imaging the peaceful place is enough to connect you with the centered state. With frequent repetition, centering and focusing can happen quickly whenever needed. You may even find that you are walking in and out of the centered state most of the time and that your work flows more easily as a result.

EXERCISE

## CENTERING

1. Working with the breath, release any heaviness, the accumulated debris of the day, worry, or concerns as you exhale. Do this three times, then ease into a very comfortable position in a chair or while laying down.

*(continues)*

*(continued)*

2.  In your mind's eye, allow yourself to go to a time when you felt very peaceful in nature. This may be a place you have visited or a picture you remember. Seat yourself comfortably and just allow yourself to enjoy the immediate moment of being in this peaceful place.

3.  See the colors around you. Notice the lighting, the shadows, the shadings of the colors. Notice the textures around you—smooth, rough, rocky, flowing. Notice clouds and other beauty. Let your awareness of this lovely place grow.

4.  Let yourself hear the sounds—a bird in the distance, the sound of flowing water, the rustle of leaves as a gentle breeze blows by.

5.  Feel the breeze on your cheeks and sense the cooling. Sense the warmth of the sun. Feel the relaxation of this peaceful place inside your body. Feel the relaxation in any areas of tension or stress.

6.  Smell the flavors of this peaceful place—the leaves on the forest floor or the fresh salt air of the sea. Enjoy all the senses as you take the inner journey to this peaceful place.

7.  Gently let your awareness shift back to the present time taking with you the feeling of relaxation and peacefulness. Know you can return to this experience whenever you choose.

## Assessment of the Biofield

After centering, you are ready to practice sensing another person's energy field. Assessment is a step that allows you to sense another's field without judgment or preconceived notions. The following exercise will help you to develop skills in assessing your client's energy field.

EXERCISE

## ASSESSING THE HEAD & SHOULDERS

1.  To begin, have a friend or interested person sit comfortably in a chair while you stand behind.

2.  Using both hands, scan above the head 1–6 inches away from the body. Sense the energy around the head, neck, and shoulders paying attention to what your hands tell you. Does the energy feel cool, warm, bumpy, smooth, or tingly? Is there a sensation of fullness, vibration, pulsation, or depletion? Do you feel pulled in or

*(continues)*

*(continued)*

pushed away? Which parts feel the same, and where are things different?

3.  Share with your friend what you noticed and ask if this has any meaning for her. If you are working with a group, it is helpful to assess another person's field in the same manner, noting how the fields of two people are similar or different.

## EXERCISE

## ASSESSING THE BIOFIELD

1.  Hold your hands above your partner's crown chakra, or the fontanel area, to discover if it feels warmer or cooler than the neck and shoulders. Hold your hands out as far as you can reach on both sides of the head and find the edge of the energy field. This edge or outer layer may extend farther than you can reach with your hands. Have your friend help you by reporting when she feels your hands in her field. Note if the field is symmetrical on both sides or distorted in some way.

2.  Work your way all around your friend's body, 1–6 inches away, noting areas of difference. The energy is smooth and symmetrical in a balanced energy field, so any differences are clues to areas of imbalance and disruption. Scan the back of the head, neck, and shoulders, following with the front of the face and neck. Standing to one side of the body, scan the chest and abdomen, then assess down the arm to the hands and down the leg to the foot. Move to the other side and repeat the assessment. From the front of the body, scan over the chest, abdomen, thighs, and calves, ending with the tops of the feet. Finally, assess the back, scanning both sides and the spine.

3.  Share the differences you noted with your friend and find out what meaning these findings have for her.

***Discussion***    It is always best to be very neutral about information you receive, letting the awareness of any meaning come from the client. There is a world of difference between saying, "I noticed some heat over the right shoulder area" and interpreting, "You have heat and congestion here that must come from too much exercise." One is simply an objective observation while the other implies judgment, likely to create defensiveness in your partner.

Sometimes your partner will make no conscious connection between what you sensed and any current symptoms. This does not mean you were inaccurate. Remember that problems appear to manifest first in the energy field before becoming identifiable physical symptoms. A pervading denial of the physical body exists in our culture, so people are often not even aware of discomfort until it is acute and above their pain thresholds. Many times people have come to us after an assessment and recalled some stress on the previous day or a prior injury that they had forgotten to mention.

Development of assessment skills requires frequent practice. Try sensing the energy of at least 20 people and notice the variations among them. Feel the head of someone who has an active headache and you will learn what this condition does to the energy field. Comparisons help you to learn differences. Is there a difference between tension, sinus, or migraine headaches? How does pain, acute and chronic, feel? Practice scanning both healthy and ill persons to help develop your sensitivity. Remembering to center first will, of course, greatly help you to increase your sensory acuity.

## Unruffling or Smoothing the Field

Unruffling, using calm and rhythmic hand movements to clear the energy field of a *ruffled* or congested area, is one of the basic healing techniques used in all healing work and described by Dr. Dolores Krieger (1993, p. 65). Unruffling may be used by itself as a simple, effective technique in any setting or in conjuction with the modulation of energy described in the next section. Unruffling requires the focused intention of the healer and allows for gradual relaxation of the healee through relief of pain, discomfort, or anxiety. Both hands are placed 1–6 inches above the client's skin in the emotional layer of the energy field. The hands are held open with the flat surface of the palm brushing down and away from above to below the problem site.

The client can be in a sitting position or lying down while the healer's hands move in the biofield, down and away from the body, utilizing either short or long connected strokes in a graceful, sweeping motion. Figure 8.2 shows unruffling in action, and the following exercise gives further detail.

When used immediately after a traumatic injury, this smoothing seems to reconnect the damaged tissue and assist the return of a normal flow of energy within the body. When unruffling, be sure to move the hands completely off the body far enough for the blockage, pain, or discomfort to drop away. This motion may be exaggerated as needed, especially if the discomfort or pain feels stuck. The purpose is to unblock the stagnated energy and to reestablish a more balanced flow in the affected body part. Unruffling may be done over a specific part of the biofield or over the entire body. In emotional depression, unruffling very often helps shift the feeling state of the patient to a more positive sense of self.

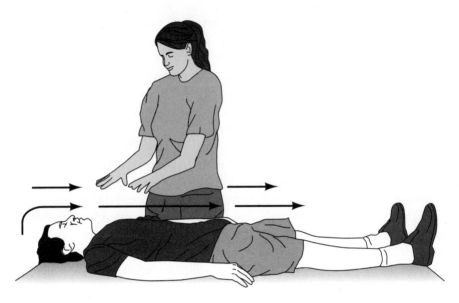

**FIGURE 8.2** Unruffling or smoothing the energy field

EXERCISE

## UNRUFFLING

1.  Select an area that is in need of smoothing or balancing from your assessment of another's energy field. (You may also ask your client or friend which physical area most needs assistance.)

2.  After centering yourself, brush away the congested area just above the skin by repeatedly sweeping with the hands from above the site to below the site.

3.  Do this for about 3 to 5 minutes noting changes in the field. Have your partner describe any sensations and share any perceptions. Look for changes in skin color, temperature, voice level, respiration, and pulse rate that come with the relaxation response and activation of the parasympathetic nervous system (Anselmo & Kolkmeier, 2000, p. 503).

## Modulation of Energy

Using the hands for the modulation of the client's energy is another basic healing technique described by Krieger (1993, pp. 70–71) and by Alice Bailey (1978, p. 649). The hands are placed directly on or slightly above the selected area of the body and held still to allow a modulation of energy from the healer to the healee. This seems to allow the client's energy to move toward balance.

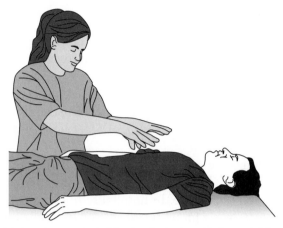

**FIGURE 8.3** The modulation of energy by holding hands above and below painful area (i.e., on foot)

The goal is to bring balance and harmony to the areas of the field that have been blocked or congested. The technique involves simply resting the hands on the specific area of the body and holding them in place for a period of time, usually 3 to 5 minutes. The hands may be kept in place until the healer feels a change, such as fullness or warmth, which is a clue that the energy has shifted.

The clues of energy change are often quite subtle: an area that was blocked and cool becomes warm; a hot area cools down; pulsation may begin; throbbing may stop; or pain may intensify, release, and quietly subside. There may be vibration, tingling, quieting, or other sensations. The healer needs to observe when change has occurred and when the specific area being treated begins to feel as symmetrical and smooth as the rest of the body (see figure 8.3).

## EXERCISE

## MODULATING ENERGY

1. With your hand scan, identify an area of the client's body that is in need of balancing, or ask your client where direct touch or modulation would be helpful.

2. After centering, place your hands directly on the identified area that has energy disturbance or pain. To work more deeply in the tissues, place the hands on opposite sides of the body. This allows a flow between your two palm chakras.

3. Hold the hands in this position for 3 to 5 minutes noting any shifts in the energy or pulsation, and listen to feedback from the client. Your hands act as the focal point of your intention and allow the client's energy to modulate toward balance.

# Closure

You may wish to reassess the field after either unruffling or modulating energy and repeat either of these processes if further balancing is needed. Recognizing when it is time to stop is the final step. Closure is indicated when there are no longer any perceivable differences in the energy field and when there is a sense of balance and symmetry. Usually, there are also shifts in the client's affect, along with deeper breathing, a flush of the skin, or other signs of relaxation that let you know when you have finished.

The client should have time to rest quietly, letting the changes integrate throughout the biofield. There is often a feeling of calmness and peacefulness. Let the client rest as long as possible. In hospital settings, the patient may drift into sleep that offers a good time for undisturbed rest. If the client needs to go to work or drive somewhere, it is helpful to take time to talk about the experience to stimulate alertness and to ensure the client is in full consciousness and safe for travel.

***Documentation*** It is also valuable to document the results of the intervention, citing what the symptoms were, the procedure used, objective and subjective observations, and feedback from the client. In addition, notice any effects of the intervention in you as the helping person, as energetic interventions can effect changes, emotionally and physically, in the healer as well.

---

**SAMPLE DOCUMENTATION OF A HEALING INTERVENTION**

| | |
|---|---|
| Presenting symptoms, and | Mrs. A. reports tightness in neck and right arm. |
| Objective assessment: | Area of heat over right shoulder, "tingling" over head and neck on energetic assessment. |
| Subjective assessment: | Mrs. A. states pain intensified during assessment. |
| Nursing Diagnosis: | Energy field disturbance, altered level of comfort. |
| Intervention given: | Smoothing biofield 10 times from top of head to below fingers, modulation by holding hands 3 minutes over right shoulder. |
| Effect: | Head, shoulder and arm have same temperature on reassessment, area feels smooth, no "tingling." Mrs. A. states she feels less discomfort, more relaxed. |

# SUMMARY

We have described four essential elements of healing interventions—centering, assessment, unruffling, and modulating energy. Each element can be used by itself, provided the healer is centered and intentional. Each process can also be used in conjunction with the other systemic and localized techniques that will be described in subsequent chapters in the next section.

# REFERENCES

Anselmo, J. and Kolkmeier, L. G. (2000). Relaxation. In Dossey, B. et al. (Eds.), *Holistic nursing*. Gaithersburg, MD: Aspen Publications.

Bailey, A. (1978). *Esoteric healing*. New York: Lucis Publishing Co.

Krieger, D. (1993). *Accepting your power to heal*. Santa Fe, NM: Bear and Co.

Nurse Healers—Professional Associates, Inc. (2000). Ziegler, J., "Report of the Coordinator," *The Cooperative Connection, XXI*:1.

Schwartz, G. & Russek, L. (1999). *The living energy universe*. Hampton, NH: Hampton Roads Publishing Co.

# SECTION III

# Healing Touch Interventions

*Throughout recorded history many teachers and healers have described techniques of working with touch. The person who wishes to be a healing practitioner usually begins learning approaches to the client's electromagnetic field by studying with someone who is an expert. The techniques are often taught by word of mouth and handed down from one generation to the next rather than being written. In the healing interventions described in this part of the book, we have attempted to include available information about the most immediate source of each intervention, but this is by no means a complete history of its origin.*

*As skill in using techniques increases, healers may blend these practices into a personal style of working directly and intuitively with the client's energy. In the next four chapters we will explore specific techniques utilized in Healing Touch and discuss considerations for developing your practice.*

# CHAPTER 9

# Full Body Techniques

*Janet Mentgen, BSN, RN*

> *"We are not interested in developing psychonoetic powers for their own sake, for the purpose of creating phenomena. We want to develop such powers only for purposes of healing, to be of service to our fellow human beings."*
>
> —Daskalos as quoted in Markides, 1987

## INTRODUCTION

As the name implies, full body techniques are used on the entire body, to complete balancing of the entire biofield. Although they usually take longer to complete than a single intervention, they have a more sustained effect. The healer uses a full body technique when there is a systemic or chronic disease process affecting the entire body. Specifically, these techniques can be utilized for toxicity, trauma, anxiety, or other systemic imbalance. A full body technique is preferred whenever there is enough time because of the greater effect on the entire field.

## FULL BODY TECHNIQUES

### Full Body Connection

The Full Body Connection has been developed from a variety of sources and is a basic technique used in the Healing Touch Program. This technique combines the concepts of the chakra connection (Joy, 1979) and chelation as taught by Rosalyn Bruyere (1989) and Barbara Brennan (1987).

To *chelate* means to claw out or to spin out. To do this, the practitioner adds a spinning motion with the hips to the hand movements given in the illustrations that follow. The spinning motion allows any heaviness, or auric debris, to spin outward with a centrifuge-like motion. This provides a more focused directing of the practitioner's intent to the client's biofield. The more intensive focus is helpful in overriding the blocks in the flow of energy that may be causing congestion or constriction in the client's biofield.

*Technique*    During this technique the client is usually lying on his back, although it can be modified to accommodate someone lying on the stomach or side or sitting in a chair. The steps of this technique are illustrated and described in the Full Body Connection exercise.

Each of the points in the technique are held from 1 to 3 minutes depending on the degree of healing and energizing work that needs to be done or on the time available. The healer stands on the right side of the patient when performing this technique. Move the lower hand to the upper hand position first in order to maintain contact with the client at all times.

*Effect*    The Full Body Connection can be used by itself or as a beginning for further interventions. While doing the procedure, the practitioner may notice areas of the biofield that seem less responsive than others. This may indicate a blocked area that may require further work. By balancing the client first with the Full Body Connection, other more specific interventions can be added later and are usually even more effective. If the procedure is used by itself, the effect may be deep relaxation or increased awareness in the client.

## EXERCISE

## FULL BODY CONNECTION[1]

The Full Body Connection may be done with the chelation, or spinning motion, by the practitioner. It can also be done by holding the hands on or over the client's body.

1.  After centering, begin by holding the sole of the right foot and the right ankle, holding until a flow occurs between your palms. You may feel movement or spinning in your own body or hands as part of the chelation. Spin your energy flow clockwise to clear this area of any congestion, fast enough to rotate the energy to

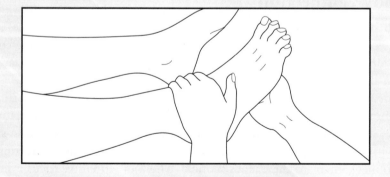

*(continues)*

---
[1] Figures reprinted with permission from Janet L. Mentgen, Program Administrator, Healing Touch.

*(continued)*

the point of release. Do this until the area underneath your hands feels full, balanced, and free, or until you cannot get any further movement.

2. Move the hands to the right ankle and knee while chelating, or spinning, your body with a clockwise rotation.

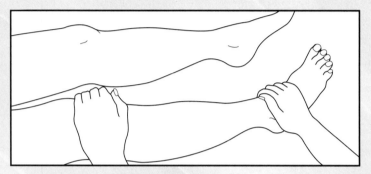

Continue the spinning of your body as you move through the following steps.

3. Move to connect the right knee and the right hip joint.

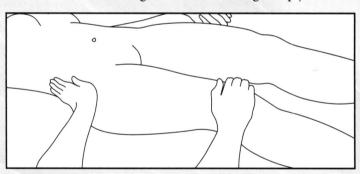

4. Reach across the body and hold between the palms of your hands the sole of the left foot and the left ankle.

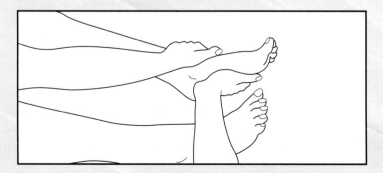

*(continues)*

*(continued)*

5. Move to the left ankle and knee.

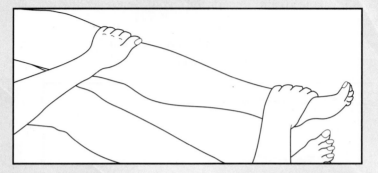

6. Hold the left knee and hip joint.

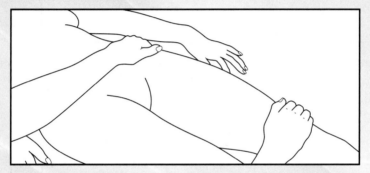

7. Hold both hip joints. At this time you may check the right and left sides of the body for balance as you sense the energy flow through the hips.

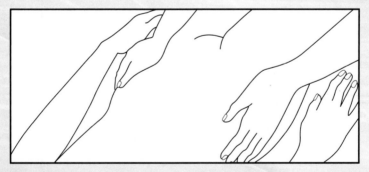

8. Place the right hand at the root chakra, between the legs about 6 inches below the floor of the perineum, or above the pubic bone, and the left hand on the sacral chakra, slightly below the umbilicus. Continue your focus on spinning your chakras as you chelate, until they match, balance, and feel equal. The best way to spin the root

*(continues)*

*(continued)*

chakra is for the healer to spin her own root chakra with a clockwise rotation and let the healee's chakra match the spin.

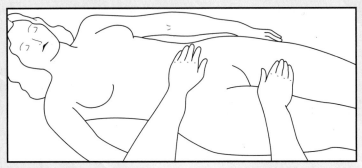

9.  Slide the lower right hand underneath the upper left hand at the sacral chakra, pause with the doubled hands for a few seconds, and then move the left or upper hand to the solar plexus center. You may notice your hands feel like they are going deeper into the body as you continue to spin your own centers.

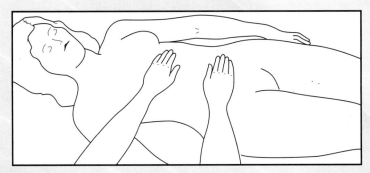

Continue to spin clockwise until the energy feels smooth and even, or until you are aware that you have held it long enough.

10. Keeping the left hand on the solar plexus move the right or lower hand to the spleen area on the left side of the body over the lower

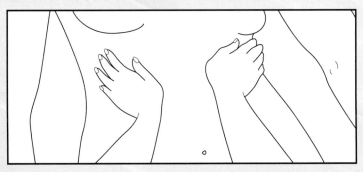

*(continues)*

*(continued)*

edge of the rib cage. Then move the left hand to the right side of the body over the liver area and spin clockwise again. Hold until there is a sense of smooth flowing and balance.

11. Move your right hand back to the solar plexus and your left or upper hand to the heart center area. Feel the hands spin downward in the spiral to match the two centers, then chelate your own body clockwise.

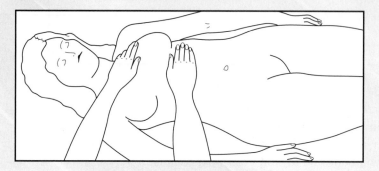

12. Using your right hand take the client's right hand and lock thumbs matching your palms together and put your left hand on the wrist. Send the energy through your palms creating a flow and continue balancing.

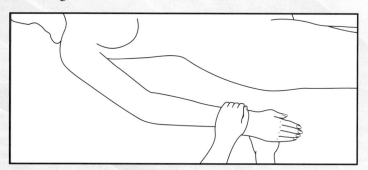

*(continues)*

*(continues)*

13. Move your hands upward to the right wrist and elbow, continuing your own chelation motion.

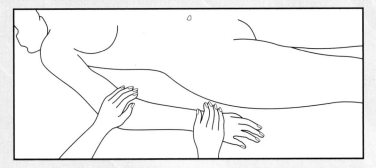

14. Hold the elbow and shoulder.

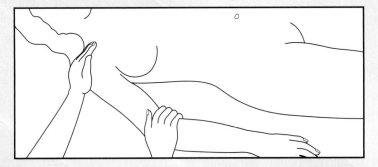

15. Reach across the body to hold the left palm and wrist.

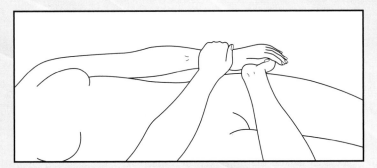

*(continues)*

*(continued)*

16. Hold the left wrist and elbow.

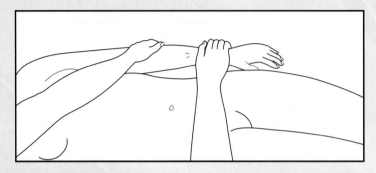

17. Hold the left elbow and shoulder.

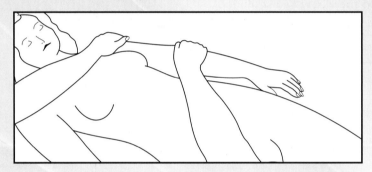

18. Hold both shoulders, again checking the right and left sides for balance, and chelate this area.

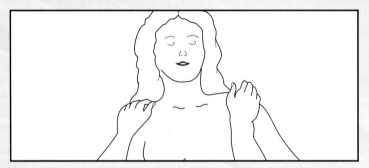

*(continues)*

*(continued)*

19. Return the right hand to the heart center and the left hand to the throat. The hand is held lightly over the notch of the neck between the collar bones. (An alternate position is to hold behind the neck with the left hand.)

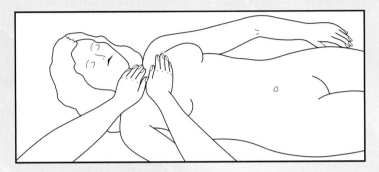

20. Bring the left hand to the brow center and move the right hand to the front of the throat.

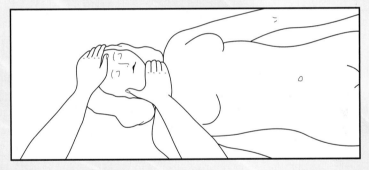

21. Place the left hand on the top of the head at the crown center with the right hand on the brow.

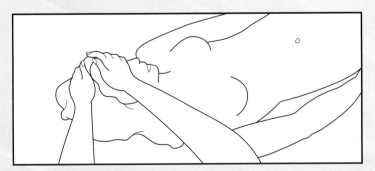

*(continues)*

*(continued)*

22. The process is completed by holding the crown with the right hand and extending the left hand straight above the crown with the palm pointed outward toward the transpersonal point that extends about 18 inches above the head.

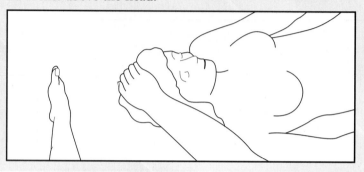

## Etheric Vitality

Etheric Vitality is a technique described by a Greek healer as a preparatory meditation for the caregiver (Markides, 1987, pp. 58–60). Labeled by Janet Mentgen, Etheric Vitality is a self-directed meditation to prepare the helper and client for relaxation and centering. This technique opens the chakra system in the healee, who may describe feeling a variety of body sensations.

Doing this meditation with the hands on the client's head is a preparation for healing interventions that follow. It is a powerful centering process as it opens the channel for connecting with the Universal Energy Flow of the healee as well as the healer.

EXERCISE

## ETHERIC VITALITY

1.  Sit or stand at the head of the table. The client should be lying supine with a pillow underneath the knees, keeping the back straight and the head flat. (This can also be done with the client sitting in a chair and the healer standing behind the chair.)

2.  Place the palms of your hands on the crown center of the client's head and hold this position for 7 to 10 minutes, or you may hold your hands in the field above the head. Feel the energy flow, sensing when the body is fully open energetically and when it is time to stop.

*(continues)*

*(continued)*

3.  With your eyes closed or opened, repeat silently to yourself, "I focus all my attention on the soles of my feet, nothing else but the soles of the feet. My entire attention is on the soles of my feet. I hold my full attention on the soles of my feet."

4.  Continuing the silent meditation, say, "Now I move the energy upward. I feel the movement to the ankles. I am aware of only the soles of my feet and my ankles, nothing else. I hold my attention on my ankles and feet."

5.  "Now I move the energy upward from my ankles to my knees. I feel the energy moving upward as I inhale and become aware of my knees, ankles, and feet. I hold in my awareness only the feeling of my knees, ankles, and feet. Nothing else enters my mind."

6.  "I again breathe the energy from the knees into the hips and feel the energy move into the hips and pelvis. I focus my attention on my legs, hips, and pelvis. Now I breathe the light energy outward and surround my entire legs in glowing white light. I feel the healing white light all around both legs and my pelvis."

7.  "I now breathe the energy into the abdomen and imagine a nebula of blue-white light swirling clockwise. I focus entirely on the nebula of blue-white light rotating clockwise in my abdomen."

8.  "I breathe the energy into my heart and imagine a nebula of rose-white light, swirling clockwise in my heart. I focus entirely on the nebula of rose-white light watching as it swirls within my heart."

9.  "I breathe the energy into my throat and imagine a nebula of orange-white light within my throat area. I watch intensely the nebula of orange-white light within my throat as it swirls clockwise. Then I watch this nebula of intense light separate and move to each shoulder then down my arms into my palms, activating my healing hands to do the work I am about to do. I imagine the white light surrounding my arms and expanding outward all around my arms and hands."

10. "I breathe the light into my head and imagine a nebula of gold-white light inside my head and expanding outward, surrounding my head until a shimmering gold-white light is all around my head and around my entire body. I remain in this shimmering gold-white light as I do the healing work."

## Magnetic Unruffle

Magnetic Unruffling is a technique that was identified by Janet Mentgen for the purpose of clearing the entire body of congested energy. It is used when there is a history of long-term prescription or recreational drug use, after anesthesia, chronic pain, trauma, breathing of polluted air, environmental sensitivities, smoking (even when the person has not smoked for a number of years), and for systemic disease. This technique cleanses the body's energy field in a systemic way. It also assists in releasing emotional debris and unresolved feelings, such as anger, fear, worry, tension, and anxiety.

Sometimes the energy will clear in the upper portion of the body and become denser in the legs and lower body. Completing each sweep from head to toe without interruption is important for this reason. Stopping to work in one area would impede the flow that cleanses the field. The goal of the Magnetic Unruffle is to completely clear the entire biofield of any accumulations or constrictions.

### EXERCISE

## MAGNETIC UNRUFFLE

1. The healee lies on the table, on his back with shoes, belt, and glasses removed and clothing comfortably loose. The healer begins by placing the hands about 12 inches above the healee's head. The fingers are spread, relaxed, and slightly curved, and the thumbs are either touching each other or close together. Use a long continuous raking motion over the entire body starting above the head and moving down the center of the body to the feet. The movement of the hands from head to toe should be in one smooth, continuous motion, uninterrupted until coming off the body beyond the toes. Continue the pull beyond the body until the sensation of energy drops away. The movement should take about 30 seconds from head to toe, going slowly enough to feel energy gather in your hands.

2. Repeat this motion from the head to beyond the feet about 30 times, or for about 15 minutes, until the energy feels smooth and even, like glass, over the entire body. An alternative is to unruffle, or smooth, the central part of the body for 10 sweeps, and then to unruffle each side with 5 to 10 sweeps, returning to the central area to complete the process. You may also work on the back in a similar fashion. Your hands may perceive a tremendous buildup of dense energy as you unruffle the biofield. A useful metaphor is to

*(continues)*

*(continued)*

imagine the hands as magnets and the debris in the energy field like iron filings that are attracted to the magnet and stick to it. Each time your hands come off the body you will need to shake or pull off the sensation of the iron filings on your hands.

3. Each stroke may feel different as new layers of the biofield clear. Visualize the layers of the field as the growth rings within a tree. Each year a new ring of the tree is created and is stored in the structure of the trunk; in a similar way, the body creates new energy layers, one by one, as we grow and change. A buildup of congested energy can occur, which may contain old memories, pain, or traumatic events. As each layer is released, the next layer emerges.

# Chakra Spread

The process described in the Chakra Spread exercise is used in hospice care for the terminally ill or for persons in severe pain because it is very gentle. Families who are sitting with a dying patient can also benefit from this technique to reduce their own stress levels.

The many applications of this technique include severe pain, before and after medical procedures, pre- and postsurgery intervention, severe stress reactions, to ease any critical life transition, and to assist someone who is choosing to enter a profound meditation. This powerful technique takes a person to a deeper level of healing than is achieved by most techniques, so its use should be reserved for special needs and sacred moments in healing.

*Technique*    Usually, the client lies on his back on a massage table or a bed. Even if the client is unable to speak, awareness of others' presence and comfort is still experienced. It is helpful to show family or friends sitting at the bedside how to hold the hand of a loved one in the locked thumb position with the other hand on top, assisting them to offer the gift of touch. A quiet environment, subdued lighting, slow relaxing music of a meditative nature assist the process. The healee may have special requests for music.

All of your movements in this technique need to be very slow and gentle, avoiding any jarring or sudden, quick movements. Remember that the patient may be very weak, severely traumatized, hypersensitive, or sedated. Any sudden movement may intensify the pain or disrupt the biofield.

With this process, pain will often diminish, or the client may relax deeply and fall asleep. After the person has relaxed completely, fears and other emotional issues that need to be processed will sometimes surface. The healer or family members need to be available for this sharing.

The technique can also be done in silence and takes about 10 to 15 minutes. It is better to repeat the technique frequently than to extend the time. Family members or caregivers can learn the procedure so relief may be offered whenever they are present. All caregivers need to do the Chakra Spread in a similar manner as familiarity and repetition provide comfort when the client is in a terminal, comatose, or unconscious state.

As a variation, the Chakra Spread may also be completed in a chair. Security is necessary because the patient may relax, fall asleep, and slip out of the chair. Begin by holding the feet and the hands. Then, go behind the chair and begin the procedure gently and slowly three times at the top of the head, the crown, brow, throat, and heart centers. Move to the front of the healee and squat or kneel to spread the chakras at the solar plexus, abdomen, root, hips, knees, and ankles. Pull the energy off the tops of the feet. Repeat the sequence three times and end by holding one hand while placing the other hand on the heart.

## EXERCISE

## CHAKRA SPREAD

1. After centering, begin by holding the sole of the foot with the palm of your hand and place the other hand on top of the foot or ankle. Hold for at least a minute to open the energy center at the sole of the foot as a release for pain, tension, or anxiety. Hold the other foot in like manner for a minute.

2. Go to one side of the patient and hold the hand by locking thumbs, with your palm touching the client's palm and placing your other hand on the back of the patient's hand. Hold for at least a minute to open the energy flow in the palm chakra, creating a drain or release for accumulated stress. Repeat this hold on the other hand.

3. Move to the top of the head and bring both hands together into the energy field above the crown chakra. You will feel the edges of the chakra as you enter the field. Gently and slowly spread both hands outward as far as you can reach. Repeat this three times.

4. Spread each lower chakra in similar fashion in the following order: crown, brow, throat, heart, solar plexus, abdomen, and root chakra. Notice how each chakra area feels. Continue by spreading the energy areas around the knees and the ankles.

5. Pull the energy off each foot by placing one hand above the foot and one hand below the sole of the foot. The pulling away resembles bringing a column of light off the foot.

*(continues)*

*(continued)*

6. Return to the crown and repeat the spread on each chakra 3 more times.

7. Repeat this sequence one more time, completing three entire rounds.

8. To complete the technique, return to one hand of your client and hold it again in the locked thumb position while placing your other hand on the heart center area of the patient.

# Etheric Unruffle

In 1991, Rod Campbell, an Australian healer, demonstrated a technique to Janet Mentgen. She modified it and labeled the procedure Etheric Unruffling. This very simple procedure creates a profound effect by working on the etheric or vital level of the biofield which is closest to the skin in the interface between the physical body and emotional layer.

***Technique*** The healer usually sits next to the client who is lying on a bed or table. Place the hands slightly above the body and gently move the hands until you begin to feel the etheric field. Where there is disturbance or a problem you will feel a difference in the field from the smooth flow of a clear field to the turbulence or vibration of a blocked area. Work this area by moving the hands in any direction following the energetic pathways. It may feel as if you are combing the field, untangling strands, or repairing a chakra.

Etheric Unruffle teaches the healer to follow her sense of energy as a guide. Release any personal attachment to predicted outcomes, other techniques, or expectations, and simply follow the client's energy. Follow the energy by moving the hands in the client's field for an extended period of time, noting the condition and problems you encounter. Advanced Healing Touch practitioners have done this technique for longer periods of time, up to an hour, in congested or complicated fields to release energy blockage.

This is the simplest of all the techniques described. However, the development of the healer must be sufficient to understand and read the energetic response in order for this to be effective. The process is done until the energy field feels clear and smooth. It is essential that the healer be mature, centered, and attuned intuitively to the client's field.

## SUMMARY

All full body techniques have an effect on the physical as well as other layers of the biofield. The initial effect of relaxation is sometimes followed by other forms of release, such as decreased pain perception, increased mental acuity, or emotional catharsis. The increased sense of well-being may last for several days or weeks depending on the responsiveness of the client's energy system.

## REFERENCES

Brennan, B. (1987). *Hands of light*. New York: Bantam Books.

Bruyere, R. (1989, October). Workshop on energetic healing. Glendale, CA: Healing Light Center Church.

Joy, B. (1979). *Joy's way*. Los Angeles: J. P. Tarcher, Inc.

Markides, K. (1987). *Homage to the sun*. New York: Arkana Books, Penguin Group.

# CHAPTER 10

# Localized and Specific Techniques

*Janet Mentgen, BSN, RN*

> *"Thank you, my friend,*
> *For you have shared your pain.*
> *Now we can work together*
> *As we surrender to the Powers*
> *Beyond ourselves in seeking release*
> *From the twisted turbulence*
> *Within."*
>
> —Hover-Kramer, 1993

## INTRODUCTION

Specific techniques may be selected by the caregiver to accomplish specific healing outcomes. Having adequate time during an interaction with a client to find the most effective treatment is sometimes a challenge, especially in clinical settings. These guidelines are designed to help the healer select the appropriate technique quickly and to expedite the treatment of localized conditions.

## SPECIFIC TECHNIQUES

### Energetic Ultrasound

The technique we have called Ultrasound in energy healing reaches deeply into the body. Deep tissue penetration is effective for pain in arthritic joints, for stopping internal bleeding, for sealing lacerations, and for work around the eyes or ears. Ultrasound can be effective for fractured bones, tendonitis, joint injuries, and tumors. It can be used anywhere on the body where a deeply penetrating intervention is needed.

Ultrasound is always available because it requires only your hands and willingness. If we were shipwrecked on a deserted island, we could use this energetic form of Ultrasound. As one of the first aid techniques of the future, Ultrasound is effective on occasions where immediate relief from trauma is needed, establishing the process of self-healing to repair damaged tissue. The distressed pattern is broken up and reorganization of energy can occur quickly with the use of the energetic tool formed by the hand (see figure 10.1).

Animals respond to Ultrasound with immediate wound repair. Large gaping wounds woven together with Ultrasound will often shrink to a tiny scab by the next morning. Experiment to see how quickly this technique assists healing. Most Healing Touch practitioners find that repeated work with Ultrasound is even more effective than a single application.

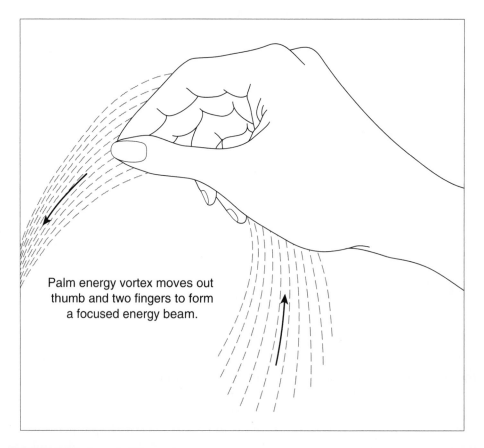

Palm energy vortex moves out thumb and two fingers to form a focused energy beam.

**FIGURE 10.1** Energetic Ultrasound.

EXERCISE

## ULTRASOUND

1. This technique is done by holding the thumb and first and second fingers together, directing energy from the palm chakra out the fingers and thumb. Imagine a beam of light coming from the fingers and thumb that is directed into the client's body.

2. Place the opposite hand behind the body part on which you are working. You can sense the beam of the light's deep penetration by feeling it in the palm of the opposing hand.

3. Try this on someone's wrist by putting one hand underneath the wrist and sending energy through the fingers and thumb of the other hand on top of the wrist.

4. To use Ultrasound, move the whole hand in any direction desired with the fingers pointed toward the area for about 3 to 5 minutes. Keep moving the hand continuously while doing Ultrasound, just as a physical therapist would move a mechanical ultrasound head.

# Energetic Laser

The Energetic Laser technique is very similar to Ultrasound. This time, one or more fingers are held still and pointed toward the problem area with the sensation of an intermittent pulsing light penetrating deeply into the tissue. Laser can be effective with isolated pain such as a toothache, TMJ (temporal mandibular joint) problems, or any situation where spot healing is needed.

The Laser can be used for cutting, sealing, or breaking up congestion. It is sometimes used with just one finger pointed directly toward the body. An alternative is to use all the fingers pointed toward each other on opposite sides of the body to intensify the intersection of energy flows and to activate a specific area within the body. The Laser appears to be very powerful and is used for only a few seconds or up to a minute.

# Mind Clearing

Mind Clearing is a technique taught by Rudy Noel, who studied extensively with Rosalyn Bruyere. Mind Clearing is used for relaxation and to focus the mind. It has become a favorite technique of Healing Touch students over the years. Family members can be taught this technique, and it is ideal for sharing in a relationship because it cannot be done easily on oneself.

*Technique*    For Mind Clearing the client is lying on his back, away from the headboard of a bed so the head can be reached easily. The healer may be standing or sitting. This technique can also be done while the client is lying on the floor or on a massage table with the healer sitting at the client's head. Another option is for the client simply to sit on a chair with the healer standing behind. However, the best results come when the client is lying down, due to the profound relaxation induced. Hold each of the steps illustrated and described in the following exercise for 1 to 3 minutes.

The client may drift to sleep or be fully relaxed. Process any thoughts or feelings that arose during the interaction. The client may share deeper levels of awareness after the body has had an opportunity to relax in this profound way, so plan some time for this exchange.

An alternate way to do the Mind Clearing is to use the palms of the hands instead of the fingertips. The effect of this is more soothing with less deep penetration into the tissues. As before, each hold is from 1 to 3 minutes.

## EXERCISE

## MIND CLEARING[1]

1.  After centering, begin by holding the fingers lightly just above the collar bone on each side of the throat. This establishes attunement between healer and healee and begins the flow of energy.

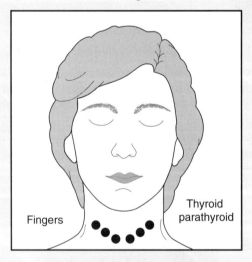

Fingers          Thyroid parathyroid

2.  Put one hand on the center of the back of the head where the skull meets the neck. Find the notch in the occipital ridge and place the middle finger in the notch. Two fingers of the opposite hand rest between the eyebrows in the middle of the forehead.  *(continues)*

---

[1] Mind Clearing sequence reprinted with permission from Rev. Rudy Noel, CET.

*(continued)*

Notice that the middle fingers will be pointing toward each other, intersecting through the midbrain. The touch is featherlight, so gentle there will be no mark of pressure left on the forehead.

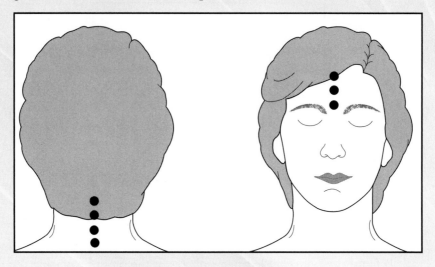

3. Place both hands under the head and wrap the fingers around the occipital ridge. Then lift the head gently with light pressure under the ridge (this usually feels good to the client). Pull the neck toward you, putting slight tension on the muscles of the neck. You may wish to ask the client if more or less pressure is needed.

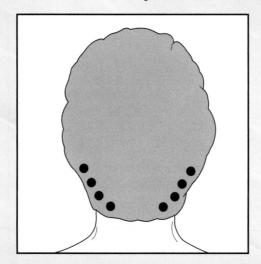

4. Hold the fingers of both hands around the skull like a cap with the thumbs on the crown of the head in the fontanel area. This point

*(continues)*

*(continued)*

on top of the head affects blood pressure, and this hold can also be used to reduce hypertension.

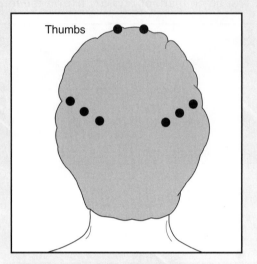

5. Balance the right and left hemispheres of the brain by placing the middle finger of each hand on a point above and slightly behind the ear at the hairline where you can feel a pulse. The pulse may feel uneven on each side at first, but with holding the pulses will move to a smooth, more balanced rhythm.

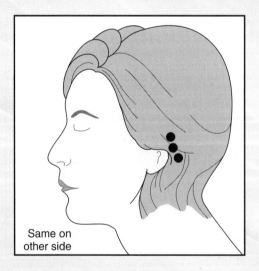

*(continues)*

*(continued)*

6. Set three fingers of each hand on a line from the inside of the eyebrows to the hairline, forming a V. Your elbows will be flared out and away from your body.

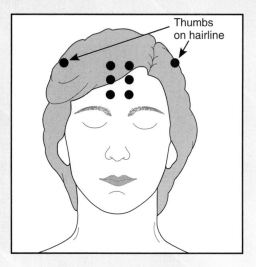

Thumbs on hairline

7. Spread the fingers to form a wider V to the outside of the eyebrow. This opens the window to the intuitive center sometimes called the third eye, and will be the peak of relaxation in the technique. The client will often experience images, dreams, colors, or deep sleep.

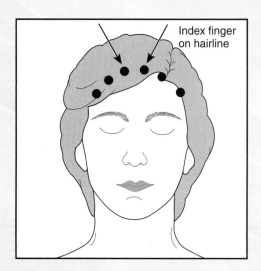

Index finger on hairline

*(continues)*

*(continued)*

8. Have the client open the mouth or yawn to help you find the mandibular joint. Then, have him close the mouth and massage this joint in the biofield by rotating your fingers using a circular motion.

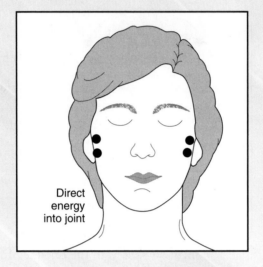

Direct
energy
into joint

9. Stroke three times from the middle of the brow, across the forehead, and down the cheeks over the mandibular joint. Add any additional gentle massage to the face and ears that seems appropriate.

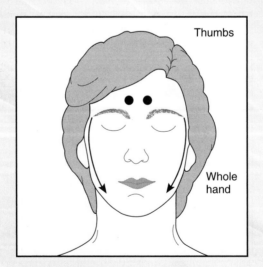

Thumbs

Whole
hand

*(continues)*

*(continued)*

10. Softly brush the cheeks with the palms, and cup the hands lightly around the jaw so the fingers point to the throat.

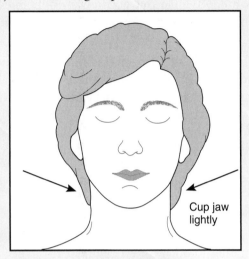

Cup jaw lightly

11. Finish with a gentle kiss, a light touch to the forehead, or a gesture, such as squeezing the shoulders, that lets the person know you are finished.

## Magnetic Pain Drain

The Magnetic Pain Drain is a useful technique for acute and painful areas as it helps to remove pain or congestion in the biofield. As in other energy-based techniques, the healer is centered, still, and attuned to the highest good of the client. The basic concept in the technique is to use the left hand as the receiver of energy and the right hand as the release or sender of energetic material. Usually, the client will relax deeply and report relief of discomfort in 3 to 5 minutes with each of the two positions described in the following exercise.

EXERCISE

## MAGNETIC PAIN DRAIN

1. Place the left hand on the area that hurts or feels congested, and hold the right hand downward and away from the body. This siphons the energy from the client's body and out the healer's right hand. The healer may sometimes feel the activity move through her body. Usually, the energy will travel into the healer's left hand,

*(continues)*

*(continued)*

up the arm, across the shoulders to the right arm, and leave the body through the hand. A pumping action with the right hand will speed up the process. Hold this position until the movement or sensation of pulling through stops and you are completely free of any pressure.

2. Reverse the hands, placing the right hand on the client's problem area and holding the left hand upward to bring in healing energy from the Universal Energy Field. This allows the void that occurred from the draining action to fill with light and warmth. Remember that any energy drained off is neutral, does not have a negative or positive quality, and quickly dissipates into the Universal Energy Field.

# Spiral Meditation

The Spiral Meditation is more fully described in *Joy's Way* (Joy, 1979) and can be utilized as a meditation to open the energy field at the beginning of a healing sequence. It is also effective as a technique for opening energy centers that are blocked or constricted in energy flow. Because of its focus on the heart center, the Spiral Meditation is also effective in strengthening the heart chakra, which is desirable if immune system function is disturbed.

## EXERCISE

## SPIRAL MEDITATION

1. With the client lying on his back, begin by placing your hands over the heart center. Following a clockwise flow, draw the spiral pattern on the full body, pausing approximately 1 minute over each energy center.

2. The sequence moves from the heart center to the solar plexus, to the high heart, down to the spleen, to the abdomen, up to the throat, then to the root, brow, knees, crown, ankles, finishing with the transpersonal point above the head.

3. Occasionally, this pattern can be modified by letting one hand follow the other hand. For example, place the right hand on the heart, and when you move the right hand to the solar plexus place the left hand on the heart, thus placing both hands on the body. The healer can also do the Spiral Meditation on herself as a self-healing process.

*(continues)*

(continued)

4.  While the spiral is open, complete any other intervention using specific or full body techniques.

5.  To complete the technique, close the spiral with a counterclockwise motion starting at the transpersonal point then moving to the ankles, crown, knees, brow, root, throat, abdomen, spleen, high heart, solar plexus, and ending at the heart center. The closing of the spiral can also be done quickly by lightly touching each point.

## Double Hand Chakra Balance

A technique to energize a specific chakra is to hold the hands, left over right, for a period of three minutes directly on the energy vortex. Starting with the root center, move to the sacral chakra below the navel; next, hold the solar plexus chakra at the pit of the stomach, and follow with the heart, the throat, the brow, and the crown. A music tape such as *Spectrum Suite* (Halpern, 1979) is useful as it plays 3 minutes of music in the musical key that matches each chakra. Add imagery to this procedure by using the color red for the root chakra, orange for the sacral, yellow for the solar plexus, green for the heart, blue for the throat, indigo for the brow, and violet for the crown center. This creates 21 minutes of deep relaxation and balances the energy centers. This is an ideal self-help process you can teach clients using a musical tape of their choice.

A supplemental Double Hand Balancing can be done on any area of the body over a minor chakra point anytime there is a need for reducing pain. If one is aware of the first signs that a center is closing down, this double hand boost can be used instantly to restore balance. Teach this simple and effective technique for clients to use on themselves daily and between visits to help strengthen their energy centers.

## Connecting the Chakras

After assessment of the energy field and the chakra system, determine which chakra needs to be energized the most. Place one hand on the selected chakra and the other hand on the chakra above it. This connects the two chakras and will bring the vibration to a higher frequency, like plugging into a storage battery. Hold the hands in place until you feel the vibrational pattern change and the energy increase, usually in 1 to 3 minutes. Continue to hold the identified chakra and move the upper hand to the next chakra above and hold until the energy stabilizes. Continue to do this until you connect the crown chakra to the identified chakra. Then work with the chakra below, connecting it in the same manner until all of the major chakras have been connected to the identified one.

For example, if you have found that the solar plexus chakra is blocked, place your right hand on the third chakra and your left hand on the fourth chakra, holding for several minutes. Then, still holding the solar plexus chakra, move your left hand to the throat center. Hold again until it feels complete, then move the left hand to the brow, then to the crown. To work down the body, continue to hold the solar plexus chakra, but with your left hand, and move the right hand to the second chakra, then to the first chakra. Each time, notice the balancing and changes that occur.

## Pyramid Technique

The Pyramid technique was shown to Janet Mentgen in meditation as a way of connecting the major chakra centers with the arms and legs. It may be done by one healer, but is even more powerful with two healers. Each position is held for 1 to 3 minutes or until the client's field is smooth and flowing.

When doing this technique with two healers, each person places a hand on the root chakra, one hand on top of the other's, and each person places another hand on the hip. This forms a dynamic triangle. Proceed through the body connecting the abdomen with the knees, the solar plexus with the ankles, the throat with the shoulder, the brow with the elbows, and the crown with the wrists. Complete with all four hands on the heart.

The Pyramid technique seems to powerfully change the energy vortices and to integrate them almost as if you were adding an electrifying current. Use this when a power boost is needed for clients with weakened conditions, fatigue, or diseases such as cancer and AIDS where the immune system is depleted. This can also be used for structural problems in the musculoskeletal system.

### EXERCISE

## PYRAMID TECHNIQUE

1.  Place the hand on the root chakra above the pubic bone and the other hand on the hip. Hold this position for several minutes, then move the hand from one hip to the other hip, leaving the hand in place on the root center. With this you are drawing a triangular configuration on the body.

2.  Move the upper hand to the abdomen, on the second chakra, and the lower hand to the knee and hold. Move the lower hand to the other knee. Notice the triangles you are creating.

3.  Move the upper hand to the solar plexus and the lower hand to one ankle and hold. Move to the other ankle and hold.

4.  Move to the upper body, placing one hand above the throat center and the other hand first on one shoulder, then on the other shoulder.

*(continues)*

*(continued)*

5. Move the upper hand to the brow center and hold the lower hand on one elbow, then on the other elbow.

6. Move the upper hand to the crown. With the lower hand hold one wrist, then the other wrist.

7. Place both hands on the heart and hold until the process of balancing feels complete.

# Lymphatic Drain

To do the Lymphatic Drain accurately, it is helpful to have a picture of the lymphatic system with you, or to remember how the system drains in the physical body. The Lymphatic Drain is a form of energetic release used to help relieve congestion and pain in the lymph system or in autoimmune diseases, such as lupus erythematosus or rheumatoid arthritis. The symptoms described by the client are generalized soreness and achiness; tenderness in the groin and neck or under the arms; and pain in the feet, ankles, and wrists.

Figure 10.2 shows the steps in numbered fashion as they are described in the Lymphatic Drain exercise. Remember to use short, brisk strokes to cleanse the energy field of congestion and follow with time for the client to rest in order to let the field realign itself.

This technique may take considerable time, from 10 to 30 minutes depending on the client's needs, but is very effective for clearing chronic and acute lymphatic congestion. It is another technique that works well with two healers working simultaneously after centering together.

## EXERCISE

## LYMPHATIC DRAIN

1. Begin by holding the fingers spread in a relaxed and raking position. You are going to drag your fingers against the etheric lymphatic layer, pulling across and down the body. Start raking on one side of the chest from the sternum and across the breast, continuing to do the short, rapid, raking motions until there is no longer any drag or thickness felt. The cleared field will feel light and flowing to the client.

2. Follow the same technique by placing the client's arms slightly away from the body and raking under the arms, then down the arms and off the fingers. These are short, quick pulling strokes, done rapidly, one section at a time.

*(continues)*

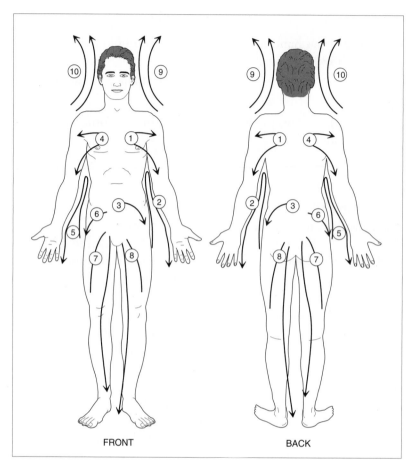

FRONT          BACK

**FIGURE 10.2** Lymphatic drain.

*(continued)*

3. Go to the abdomen and pull across the abdomen and off the body.

4-6. Go to the other side of the body and repeat the raking pattern in the chest, underarm areas, and abdomen.

7-8. Rake the area above the groin, down the legs, and off the foot. Repeat on the other side.

9-10. Go the head and rake up each side of the neck and the face to move congestion away from the head.

11. Repeat the process on the back starting with the heart area (see numbered procedure on figure 10.2).

12. Conclude by letting the client rest, allowing time for integration and any sharing.

# Technique for Sensing the Pain Ridge

When a person is experiencing acute pain, a ridge or bulge that corresponds to the pain can be found in the energetic field. This ridge may be sensed by the healer at some distance from the body, usually 12 to 18 inches away, but sometimes, as in the case of migraine headaches, it can be felt as far as 5 to 10 feet away. As you scan the field to sense the pain ridge, it usually feels warm, hot, or congested and you may sense tension or vibration in your hand.

Once you have found the ridge simply unruffle or smooth the area until it is smoothed out. Scan the energy field again, unruffling the ridge for several more minutes if needed, and then rescan. The ridge will begin to recede. Repeat this process until you can bring your hand all the way to the client's body and touch the skin without having the client report pain. This technique has been successfully used by Healing Touch practitioners on trigeminal neuralgia, TMJ syndrome, migraine headaches, and fractured bones. If the ridge persists, the Magnetic Pain Drain may also be used by placing the left hand on the pain ridge to siphon off the pain with the right hand.

# Technique for Sealing a Wound

Whenever the body has experienced trauma, has had surgery, or has given birth, the energy field, as well as the physical body, is impacted. Scan the area above the scar or injury with the palm of your hand to determine if there are any *leaks* in the biofield at the site. The leaks or breaks in the field may feel like a column of cool air, as if you are feeling a leaking inner tube. A clue that a leak is present is when a client describes a scar as remaining sore or tender for years after injury or surgery. Another symptom is a continual feeling of fatigue following a traumatic or surgical experience.

To determine whether there is such an energetic hole, check any old incisions, drainage points, or puncture sites by assessing with a hand scan. To seal the leak, gather energy from the field around the area by moving your hands with the palms toward the client's skin area, back and forth over the identified spot. Then seal this extra energy supply to the skin with the palm of your hand and hold for a minute. The sealing may sound like plastic touching a hot plate with a hiss. After the area is sealed, rescan to see if any other leaks can still be detected. The area should feel as smooth and balanced as the rest of the body.

# SUMMARY

Numerous interventions used by the healer during energy-based work are spontaneous and seem to be directed or guided, happening at an appropriate moment. Sometimes the intervention comes as an inner voice speaking to you, emerges as an image, or feels as if your hands are being pulled unexpectedly to a specific area of the healee's body. At other times, you may try to remove your hands and the magnetic pull is so great that it is almost impossible to lift them. So you remain awhile longer, holding the area until the hands can move freely. You may also feel intuitively drawn to sweep the area with unruffling of the energy field or placing hands on the area. The important thing is to listen to this inner wisdom and to observe the outcomes.

All of the techniques described in this chapter lend themselves to precise intervention for specific client needs in almost any setting. Usually, 15 to 20 minutes is ample time to do one or several of these processes in combination. The healer needs the knowledge and skill to center, plan, implement, and evaluate the procedure. All of the techniques can be done with the client fully clothed and in a variety of clinical situations. Thus, the Healing Touch interventions offer a useful complement to other treatments the client is receiving and can be integrated unobtrusively into many helping endeavors, as we shall see in section IV.

# REFERENCES

Halpern, S. (1979). *Spectrum suite*. Belmont, CA: Halpern Sounds.

Hover-Kramer, D. (1993, March). A nurse's meditation. *Journal of Holistic Nursing, XI* (1), 115–116.

Joy, B. (1979). *Joy's way*. Los Angeles: J. P. Tarcher, Inc., 191–196.

# CHAPTER 11

# Specific Interventions for Identified Problems

*Janet Mentgen, BSN, RN*

> "...*The expert will work with both the physical changes and the information's energy pattern to relieve its constriction and to assist healing the information that led to the problem.*"
>
> —Slater, 2000

## INTRODUCTION

Energy-based interventions are a complement to the client's selected medical care and support the healing abilities of the body. One important aspect of energy work is the enhanced effect of medication and chemicals within the body. The client and healer should be alert to the possibility of side effects and sensitivity reactions. Reduction of medication to lower dosages is sometimes indicated.

Selected specific interventions are presented here that can be used for physical problems. This list is not exhaustive, but it suggests some beginning energetic approaches. Because each client's energy field is unique, you may develop your own ways of working after assessing and careful attention to intuition. This information is based on the experiences of many nurse healers and can assist you, the caregiver, when you are deciding which way to approach a client with specific health issues.

## TECHNIQUES FOR IDENTIFIED PROBLEMS

### Arthritis

Use a full body technique such as Magnetic Unruffle or Full Body Connection because of the systemic nature of all arthritic problems. Follow this with Ultrasound to the specific joints involved, and teach the client how to use this technique on affected joints. The intention is to reduce pain and swelling, to retard the degenerative process, and, if possible, to restore the joint to optimum functioning.

# Back Problems

A series of steps are used for back problems that begin with an assessment of the client's biofield on the front of the body, followed by a Full Body Connection. The client is then assisted to lie prone on a massage table, preferably with a head cradle to keep the spine and neck straight. This creates a relaxed position to support further work on the back. Another option would be for the patient to lie on her side if the prone position is too uncomfortable.

The healee with acute back pain may need to be treated daily, along with other medical or complementary interventions, until the biofield of the back remains open and flowing. Treatment can be extended to every other day, and then, be given weekly until the symptoms are gone or further intervention of another kind is implemented. You will usually see the client on a weekly basis for chronic conditions.

*Assessment*   A hand scan or assessment with a pendulum determines the energy pattern, starting at the bottom of the spine. The pendulum should rotate clockwise up the entire back, at each vertebra. Note the direction and size of the spin. A disturbance or block is indicated when the pendulum does not move or is moving at an angle other than the clockwise spin. Sometimes, the pendulum will show no motion over the entire back, denoting severe blockage.

Scan the back with the hands and feel the other layers of the field, noting changes in sensation such as heat, tingling, suction, or pressure. Then visually scan the back of the patient by standing at the foot of the table. Note the length of the legs and any asymmetry in the shape of the shoulders and hips. Look at the position of the body, noting where it is straight or crooked. Visually scan from the head to the feet noting any imbalance between the right and left sides.

*Connecting the Lower Part of the Body*   The next step is to connect the back chakras of the legs by doing a partial Full Body Connection. Starting on one leg, hold the sole of the foot with the palm of one hand and the ankle with the palm of the other hand. This creates a connection of the healer's hands with the patient. Hold this position until you feel the energy flowing, pulsating, or equalizing. Then connect the ankle to the knee and the knee to the hip. Complete the other side in a similar manner, and then hold one hand on each hip. It may take a minute or two for the energy to flow and become even. Notice any differences between the legs, including movement, muscle tension, energy flow, and temperature.

*Opening the Spinal Energy Flow*   Open the spinal energy flow by placing one hand at the base of the patient's neck and the other hand at the base of the spine. The energy will move in a wavelike motion, back and forth, like a bubble in a level, which you can sense with your hands. Keep holding this position until the energy flows smoothly and evenly. In severe imbalance, you may observe that there is no response or flow of the energy, which means that other back techniques may be more effective or that additional treatment modalities are needed before the body can respond energetically.

***The Vertebral Spiral Technique***    The muscles of the spine are addressed by drawing clockwise and counterclockwise circles above the spinal column beginning at the base of the neck. With the first two fingers and thumb held together, simulate the Ultrasound effect by pointing toward the spine and circling rapidly at least 10 to 12 times over each vertebral space. At the end of the rotations over each vertebral space, the energy will collect in the palms of your hands. You can pull your hands away from the body to release the energy buildup. Taking the hands away also allows the client's energy field to reorganize itself.

The Vertebral Spiral Technique may be done by physically touching the back or working in the biofield 1 to 3 inches off the back. The effect is calming and relaxing to the small muscles that lie next to the spinal column. Work all the way down the spine alternating from right side to left side, to the coccygeal area with your spins.

***Identifying Specific Vertebrae to Release Blockage***    Use the hand scan along each vertebra to locate any further blocks or problems. Do this several times to identify the specific vertebra where energy blockage occurs. If you find the energy of the back is now flowing smoothly and the pendulum shows continuous clockwise circles, the problem was probably muscular in nature and relaxation of the back muscles was sufficient. If energy blocks are still present, then proceed with the next techniques in the specific identified areas.

***The Hopi Technique***    The Hopi Technique from the Native American tradition has been taught in the apprentice manner for many centuries.

## EXERCISE

## THE HOPI TECHNIQUE

1.  Place three fingers of each hand on either side of the spine, opposite each other at the identified spot where the blockage occurs (see figure 11.1). Rest your hands together as this keeps the energy frequency running evenly. Your fingers are pointing downward into the spine, so that the energy pours from the fingers in a laserlike fashion into the spinal column. The fingertips need to be firm on the back, and the client may feel some pressure.

2.  Hold the fingers in place letting energy flow from the fingertips into the back until pulsing occurs. Wait for a smooth, balanced feeling. There may be considerable vibration and your hands may

*(continues)*

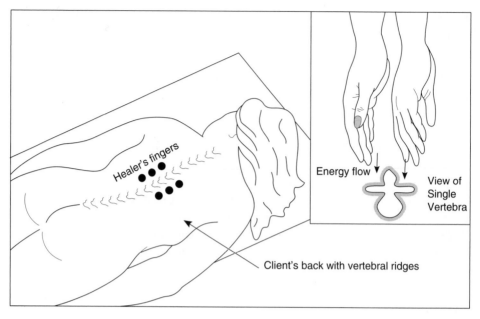

**FIGURE 11.1** The Hopi Technique, step one.

*(continued)*

shake. The key is to hold and simply stay with the vibration until it calms and becomes a gentle pulsing sensation.

3.  Place both thumbs on one side of the spine closest to you and all the fingers of both hands on the opposite side of the spine as illustrated in figure 11.2. This forms an energetic ring as the etheric extensions of your fingers wrap around the spine. The energetic fingers will extend and sink inside like a claw to wrap around the specific area of the spinal column.

4.  Have the client breathe deeply and experience any inner sensations and emotions. Images, such as events of the initial injury, may appear to the client. The client may feel pain, discomfort, movement, or heat. Wait until the energy intensifies and pulsates. Breathe rhythmically with the client to establish a slower pace. When the energy connection is complete and the spine feels balanced, pull the hands rapidly straight up, breaking through the many layers of the biofield.

5.  Reseal the field by placing both hands over the area of the back on which you were working. The client often feels the intensity of the energy connection and may have a sensation of temporary pressure or discomfort, which is followed by a physical or emotional release.

*(continues)*

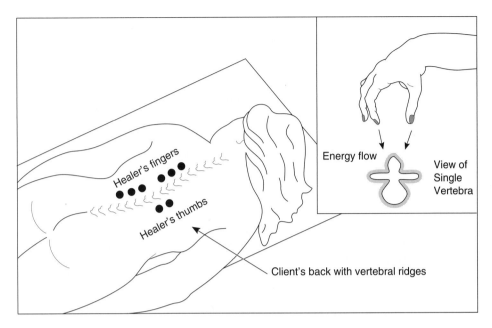

Energy flow

View of
Single
Vertebra

Healer's fingers

Healer's thumbs

Client's back with vertebral ridges

**FIGURE 11.2**   The Hopi Technique, step two.

*(continued)*

6. The healer can now work on other blocked areas of the back as identified by scanning. Sometimes one release will affect the whole back, and sometimes each individual area requires the Hopi Technique.

***Repairing Nerve Damage***   If there has been nerve damage, indicated by radiating pain following a nerve track, it is helpful to use the Laser or Ultrasound techniques by following the entire nerve. Knowledge of neuroanatomy is helpful, as well as having a mental picture of the neurological system while you are working.

***Ultrasound to Repair Muscles and Joints***   Ultrasound can be used on muscles and joints where pain is experienced. Often pain is referred and dependent from a spinal area; for example, the side of the hip may hurt from an energy block in the back. Always trace the entire pain track if possible.

***Magnetic Pain Drain***   The Magnetic Pain Drain described in chapter 10 is also effective in working with painful areas of the back.

***Sweeping and Closing***   On completion of the back techniques, close by placing one hand on the top of the neck and the other hand on the base of the spine. Then, holding one hand at the top, brush or sweep down and away several times to smooth the field. Have the client rise slowly and carefully. Since the energetic changes in the back take a while to be felt, wait for at least 24 hours before evaluating results of the treatment.

***Focusing on the Meaning of Back Problems***    The back and neck are areas in which emotional issues are often stored. These need to be examined along with the physical symptoms. Common expressions about the back in our vernacular refer to emotional states. For example, we speak of feeling "straight-backed," "flexible," "stubborn," "stiff-necked," "having our back up," "carrying a cross on the back," "sticking one's neck out," "getting ahead of oneself," "looking back," "feeling backed into a corner," or "holding back." The sense of wanting to be "backed up" can represent the need for emotional, financial, or physical support. Even if you are not trained in emotional therapy, you have a responsibility to help the client explore these insights and to refer your client to appropriate practitioners for further treatment of psychological issues.

# Neck Problems

Neck techniques are very similar to the procedures described for the back but require a finer and lighter touch. Remember that healing happens in the energetic body rather than by physical positioning or manipulating. With muscle relaxation the vertebrae will sometimes reposition themselves, but the goal of these techniques is the balancing of the energy field.

Begin by asking the client to relax the body and find a position in which you can comfortably reach the neck. Keeping the neck and head straight is important for energetic work. After assessing the neck to identify areas of blockage, use the Vertebral Spiral Technique over the seven small neck vertebrae. Reassess and if necessary follow with the Hopi Technique. Specific techniques, such as repairing nerve damage, Ultrasound, and Magnetic Pain Drain, may be used as indicated, followed by a complete brushing or sweeping of the energy field.

# Fractured Bones

A systemic intervention, such as the Full Body Connection or Magnetic Unruffle, is helpful after any trauma to restore the balance and flow of the energy field. Use Ultrasound and unruffling over a fractured bone. Sometimes, a Laser beam into the specific area will also be helpful.

***Bone Healing***    The fastest bone healing witnessed by the author occurred in 48 hours, and was confirmed by X ray. The patient was treated immediately after a fracture of the humerus, midway down the arm, with 6 minutes of unruffling and Ultrasound while she was standing under a shower. She experienced very little pain and was only inconvenienced by the wearing of a splint for a week to be assured the bone was healed.

Another example was a home care client with a fractured tibia from osteoporosis that healed in 3 months. The ankle was not casted due to severe swelling and limited mobility of the patient. Codeine was used for pain control. Ultrasound to the fracture site and Full Body Connection were used 2 to 3 times a week by several home health caregivers.

A Healing Touch practitioner witnessed an unusual healing with her son who sustained a compression fracture of the back. The tips of the vertebrae at T-10, T-11, and T-12 were knocked off and could be seen floating free from the spine on X ray. He was treated with a back brace, which he wore faithfully for 2 weeks, and pain medication, of which he took only one dose. In addition, unruffling was done on his back 3 to 4 times daily for the first 2 weeks. Then he was pain-free except for occasional back strain. After he joined the Navy, he was questioned about his fractured back, as evidenced from medical records. He showed no scarring or evidence of fracture on repeated X ray. Amazingly, not only were the tips of the bones back in alignment, but no scar line was visible on later X rays.

## Multiple Sclerosis (MS)

People with MS or other demyelinating symptoms are unable to maintain an open energy system. The energy centers will open easily with a Full Body Connection, but they will not stay open. From our experience, it takes nearly 6 months of weekly balancing by the therapist and daily work by a family member to help the energy field to maintain a full and open flow. Symptoms seem to disappear in reverse order, with the most recent symptom disappearing first. There is usually steady but subtle improvement. Keeping written records of the release of symptoms is important in order to measure progress over such a long period of time.

Balancing the field seems to enhance any other practices the client is already doing. Energy interventions may slow down the degenerative process of the disease. The difficult part, as mentioned, is the continued repetition that is required to maintain an open field. It is helpful to teach a family member or friend to use the Full Body Connection and Magnetic Unruffle on a daily basis. Additional therapeutic interventions of imagery, focusing, and psychotherapy are also helpful.

## Premenstrual Syndrome (PMS)

In persons who suffer from PMS the entire chakra system seems to go into spasm at a specific time in the menstrual cycle. Once there is a spasm, a biochemical process follows, which produces the systemic premenstrual symptoms. After the initial closing of the energy field, most treatments seem only to chase symptoms. To work with the energetic spasm, daily scanning and recording of the condition of each chakra is needed to identify specifically when a chakra shuts down so that it can be energized immediately. It may take several months of observation to determine the client's pattern.

To assist the client, balance the body fully every week with the Full Body Connection or the Double Hand Chakra Balance. The client learns to sense how an open and balanced chakra system feels and develops ways of sensing when the chakras close. After 3 to 4 months of self-observation, the client can usually identify specifically when the chakras close, which one closes first, and the specific time when this occurs. For example, the client may precisely state, "At 10:30 a.m. on day 19 of the cycle, the throat chakra closes. On day 20, three more are closed, and on day 22, I experience the systemic symptoms of bloating, irritability, and achiness." If the beginning of the energetic spasm is caught immediately, the complex symptoms of PMS may be prevented and the client can become asymptomatic.

# Headaches

To work on a headache, the most common symptom of pain in our society, first identify the type of headache with which you are working. A careful history will be helpful to determine the pattern, frequency, intensity, duration, medications, and treatments used for relief.

***Tension Headaches***    Tension headaches are muscular in nature, and usually originate in the upper or lower back and involve the back of the neck and head. The techniques of Full Body Connection, Mind Clearing, and Magnetic Unruffle are helpful to eliminate the pain.

***Sinus Headaches***    Sinus headaches, due to allergies, irritations, and infection, create frontal pain and may require medication as well as energy work. Direct release by balancing the crown, brow, and throat chakras, followed by Ultrasound and unruffling, seem to be most helpful. This can be repeated frequently until symptoms abate. Decongestive medication may interfere with the symptomatic relief and immediate results may be less evident, but it is wise to offer Healing Touch treatments as an adjunct to medications and to enhance the effectiveness of medications.

***Migraine Headaches***    Migraine headaches require a specific treatment protocol. The client should be seen weekly for a Full Body Connection and to obtain a complete history of the headache pattern. If you see the client during an acute headache, unruffle the pain ridge, which can only be done in the acute phase. This ridge often has a spike that is in the direction of the headache and can be sensed many feet away from the body. Note how the pattern of the headache begins to change and eventually stops with continued energy-balancing work. Unfortunately, most pain medication used for migraine headache relief closes the chakras and related layers of the energetic field blocks neuroreceptor sites for endorphin production.

***Head Trauma***    Head trauma responds best to the Full Body Connection, the Etheric Unruffle, and the Magnetic Unruffle. Repair the trauma site and the energy field around the head to restore the shape of the etheric field. Closed head injury symptoms respond with energy balancing techniques, such as Mind Clearing, over a period of 3 to 4 months.

## Hypertension

The person with hypertension usually has a blocked root chakra, and the Full Body Connection is the most helpful treatment. If the person remains on anti-hypertensive medication, it takes about 6 weeks before a measurable decrease in the blood pressure is noted. If the person is not medicated, there is often an immediate, measurable response of blood pressure drop during the energetic treatment. To work successfully with blood pressure reduction over the long term, encourage the lifestyle changes needed in addition to weekly energy balancing and self-care techniques. Lifetime monitoring of blood pressure is recommended. Many healers also use biofeedback tapes and relaxation training as additional therapies.

# PRE- AND POSTOPERATIVE TECHNIQUES

Prior to surgery, see the patient for energetic balancing and relaxation training. The more prepared the person is for the surgical intervention, the easier the surgical experience usually is. It makes a significant difference if the client enters the surgical procedure in a relaxed and balanced state, rather than in a tired, stressed, or fearful condition. Relaxation can happen very rapidly with the Full Body Connection or Magnetic Unruffle.

Instruct the client to tell the anesthesiologist that he is working with energetic approaches and may require less anesthesia. This is to prevent toxicity from over-use of medication. Also, encourage the patient to request having meditation tapes in the operating and recovery rooms and to limit all conversation to positive suggestions for healing. Remember that the unconscious mind hears and takes in literally everything that is said in the surgical arena.

The hospital staff may not understand or be supportive of these approaches, mostly due to lack of knowledge. It is the patient's right to have what he wants in the hospital setting, which includes an environment that is conducive to healing.

Postoperatively, the patient needs to be balanced fully to restore the energetic flow and to release any of the anesthesia trapped in the cellular tissues. Use the Magnetic Unruffle to release the chemicals, smooth the energy over the surgical site, and then gather energy for sealing the wound. Seal any puncture holes in the skin and do not forget the holes in the energy field left by drainage tubes. Energize the IV bottle and solution by holding your hands around the bottle and tubing, and energize all medication and dressings with your hands and your intention.

Teach the patient how to unruffle the site before blood is drawn and to unruffle any area where IM or IV medication is injected. Nausea is helped by unruffling and balancing the solar plexus chakra.

## Pain Control

For pain control, instruct the client in self-care techniques, such as unruffling or moving the energetic Ultrasound around painful areas. Discuss how the patient can ask for pain medication if needed and how to refuse medication if it is not needed. Hospital personnel sometimes medicate using protocols for the general public rather than addressing the individual needs of the patient. Family members can help by using the Chakra Spread for relaxation, applying the Pain Drain for pain relief, and by massaging the feet.

# MEDICAL PROCEDURES

Here are some simple hints to help reduce pain and anxiety before, during, and after invasive medical procedures. Before inserting a nasogastric tube, unruffle the throat area and make sure you as the caregiver are centered. Before beginning an intravenous infusion, unruffle over the site to be punctured. The vein will not roll, will stand up nicely for you, and the procedure will not cause pain. To remove a needle, unruffle the area as you hold the site with cotton and pressure. Smooth or unruffle any treatment site to relieve pain and help medication to absorb more readily. Modulate energy from the Universal Energy Field to assist the patient at any time during a procedure by simply placing the hands on or above the procedure site.

# SUMMARY

As can be seen, there are numerous direct applications of Healing Touch for medical problems. There is not sufficient space to go into all of them in detail, but this presentation gives you some ideas about ways to begin. As you find an approach that is helpful to the client, other techniques and intuitive ways of working with the client's biofield will often come to you.

The rapid relaxation that occurs with the energy-based techniques allows you as the caregiver to be genuinely present to assist the patient. The emotional impact of these interventions is increased trust and rapport between the caregiver and the client. And, patients are often delighted to find that they can participate in preventing their own discomfort. This sense of self-control and mastery of the environment is often a most significant outcome because patients and staff alike are trying to cope with the impersonal, mechanized settings that characterize most hospitals and out-patient clinics.

# REFERENCE

Slater, V. (2000). Energetic healing. In Dossey, B. et al. (Eds.), *Holistic nursing*. Gaithersburg, MD: Aspen Publishers, 188.

# CHAPTER 12

# The Clinical Practice of Healing Touch

*Janet Mentgen, BSN, RN*

*"Healing Touch is the art of caring that comes from the heart of the healer and reaches to the person who is receiving help."*

—Janet Mentgen

## INTRODUCTION

Healing happens within the client as the energy system establishes a state of energetic balance. From an energy-based perspective, physical or mental disease is understood as imbalance or disharmony in the client's entire energy field. It is the work of caregivers and health care professionals to assist in the restoration of balance. This is accomplished by creating a healing environment and by facilitating connection with the client's own healing potential. The outcome of an intervention from a helper may be full restoration of balance in the field, partial regaining of balance (which means accepting some areas of imbalance), or physical death with the possibility of expansion in the other dimensions of the energy field.

A healer must trust that what occurs in this subtle, noninvasive work is for the highest good of the individual. The energy that the healer helps to make available will be used in the way that is most appropriate for the client. This means that we do not really know what the best outcome would be from our limited perspectives and that we must learn to operate from the larger picture that includes the client's inner world. We always heal from the place of neutral detachment, letting go of any personal attachment to outcomes. This does not mean withdrawal or indifference but rather a state of being centered and fully present, while releasing personal investment in the client's choice or path. We learn to help as we can, and to leave without comment so that the healing process can unfold without interference. This allows the wisdom of the client's inner healing power to emerge.

In this chapter we will explore the qualities and development of the healer that allow this kind of practice to happen. We will further discuss how the healing environment can be established and will delineate the steps of a Healing Touch treatment sequence.

# THE HEALER

## Attributes of a Healer

The healer's intent is to help someone in need and to see the person in wholeness. This means that there is a sense of commitment and focus on what is best for the client. The response of the healer becomes automatic in situations of need and may range from performing an actual Healing Touch procedure to simply imaging the client in health while sending the pure intent of caring. There are truly hundreds of opportunities to assist others when we are open and flexible.

The healer's ability to center is essential. Centering is the focused intent that is required to hold a point of reference, which is the connection with the soul and the Universal Energy Field through the head, heart, and hands. In addition, the healer's physical body needs to be relaxed, the emotions calm, the mind clear of tension, and the spirit quiet and still. Thus, maintaining a personal state of wellness and vitality and minimizing stresses whenever possible becomes the ongoing preparation of the healer.

Other qualities of the healer include spontaneous compassion for the client, a sense of self-confidence, trust in the resources of the Universe, and a firm knowledge and skill base. The abilities to use imagery, to guide others, and to creatively bring ideas together are other helpful attributes. As we develop these essentials and share with our clients, there is a sense of joy and personal satisfaction.

## Development of a Healer

How does one learn to be a healer? There is often an identifiable learning sequence. It may begin with a life event, a loss or a serious illness that drives us into new ways of thinking. Our personal experience becomes a great teacher; the perceived crisis becomes an opportunity for stretching and exploring new possibilities. As we open with increasing curiosity to whatever presents itself, we notice what works and what does not to facilitate the restoration of health and harmony. Then, we move beyond our personal boundaries to apply what we have learned in helping others.

***The Choice***    The choice to work in one of the healing arts may be made consciously after resolving a personal crisis, or it may be made subconsciously out of the desire to heal oneself. Many people in the healing professions today experience frustration in their work because they are unable to fully express their creative wish to help others. Another part of the frustration among health caregivers comes from unresolved personal issues that may have attracted us to becoming helpers early in life.

To become a genuine healer means making a serious commitment to self-knowledge and compassion for others. In other words, the choice to work in a health-related field is merely a beginning. Facing one's doubts, fears, past traumas, and personal shadow is part of the development needed. Self-awareness and confidence also protect the client from misguided projections and assist the healer to set clear boundaries and stay unobtrusive. Learning to be a healer, then, requires development of oneself with experience, openness, and discipline. We will deal more fully with the vital issues of self-care and personal growth of the healer in section IV.

***Study*** Healing work demands diligent study of the art and science of healing. Knowledge of anatomy, physiology, the emotional and mental dimensions, social and medical science, intuition, counseling, and a personal sense of spiritual connection are all essential. There is literally no end to the information we can gather, or the classes we can attend, to become proficient in assisting others. Fortunately, we do not have to wait to be an accomplished expert. We grow with the process of questioning and exploring, initially learning from other healers who have the expertise, and then letting our own experience become the teacher and guide.

***Practice*** In addition to studying, you may begin to practice with family members, friends, animals, and plants before tackling strangers and patients. No matter how awkward the beginning, practice, practice, and more practice is essential to sense energy in your hands. Practice feeling the energy fields around others, sick or well, in order to identify how human energy responds. Practice sensing the biofield whenever anyone calls your attention to pain, discomfort, injury, or emotional distress, and you will quickly learn to differentiate a pain-free field.

Most important is the intuitive knowing to pause, listen, and respond before taking any action. Healers spend much time learning to be fully in the here and now, in the moment, when the world stops and opens to the present. Awareness of clients' needs comes from being fully present and attuned. Then, your body quickens, like an antenna going up and rotating in all directions to pick up the cues. Only after this careful attuning do you move into action. You can proceed without doubt; you know intuitively just what to do. Sometimes you are drawn to a location in a client's energy field without cognitive perception. It is as if you are guided to do the healing work once you have paid attention to all the preparatory steps.

# CREATING A HEALING ENVIRONMENT

It is not easy for a person who is in pain or experiencing fear to trust that physical or emotional sensations can be released. The distress of serious illness, or panic from loss of control of the physical body, can cause frustration, disappointment, and discouragement, creating severe tension. The work of the healer is to help establish an environment that assists the client to experience relaxation in the body, to release emotional attachments and the need for control, to develop an attitude of hope, and to surrender to higher guidance or inner knowing.

Ideally, the healing environment is one of simple beauty that encourages feelings of safety and protection. This may not always be possible in health care settings, so it is even more important to build rapport through your caring, gentleness, honesty, and support. Enter the client's energy field with softness, as any rough or quick movement is jarring and may create more pain and discomfort. For the client, receiving your touch is like being held, rocked, and caressed. This kind of sensation allows the client to surrender so that energy repatterning toward wholeness can happen. Healing begins when the client's body rebuilds itself because no tension or blockage stands in the way. This can happen best when the healer is centered and the healee is relaxed.

Observers are often present, such as students, family, or other professionals. As the healer and healee center and attune, the awareness of others seems to disappear. The more experienced you are, the less self-conscious you will feel about doing Healing Touch with others present. Another option is to invite the observers to add their centering, interest, intent, and caring to the effectiveness of the work.

As already implied, the work must be done in an atmosphere of trust. The healer learns to trust his inner, subtle perceptions; the client trusts the knowledge and skills of the healer; they both trust that the appropriate outcomes will emerge. Confidentiality is, of course, essential.

# HEALING TOUCH SESSIONS

Although many Healing Touch interventions can be given in a few moments in busy hospital settings, the ideal is a 1-hour healing session that can be scheduled privately at the client's convenience. By following a plan such as the one outlined here, you will be able to work in an organized way. Documentation of the interventions used also assists treatment planning, especially if the client comes several times. Needless to say, all client records must be kept secure and private in a locked filing system.

# Steps in Healing Touch Sessions

***Initial Interview***   The initial interview provides the working base for energetic interventions and functions as an intake assessment. A data sheet is needed to record enough information about the client's initial status to make effective comparisons later. You will find a sample intake sheet in Appendix D.

The first contact with the client is an important occasion. Introduce yourself and explain enough about your work so that a feeling of confidence can begin to develop. Determine the reasons the client has come, asking for data about the problem. All data you collect about the client assists you in determining the energetic patterns. To this end, relevant medical history, hospitalizations, diseases, injuries, and diagnoses, as well as medication history, are helpful. Ask about current medications, including recreational drugs, alcohol, caffeine, nicotine, vitamins, and herbs, as their ingestion may significantly impact the energy field.

It is helpful to determine which layer of the field is most important to the client's self-perception so that your treatment plan can directly address the needs of the client. The client's most perceived concerns may be in the physical, emotional, mental, or spiritual dimension or in a combination of dimensions. The client may speak of feeling "scattered," "dense," "spacy," "together," or use metaphorical expressions, like "I've been dragging around," "I feel pushed," or "I'm getting ahead of myself." These phrases of speech give clues to current stresses in the personal or professional life that you can further explore.

Look at major issues in lifestyle, relationships, perceptions, and goals. Over time, stress can build to cause repeated deficits in the energy field and the onset of physical symptoms. It is also useful to find out which areas of the person's life are going smoothly. Information about relaxation and play will tell you how the client nurtures himself and paces his lifestyle and awareness to self-caring activities. In the current time of public interest in self-improvement, many clients come with experience in support groups, self-hypnosis, meditation, 12-step programs, imagery, daily exercise, and nutritional planning. All of the activities the client is already doing can become valuable resources as you plan your interventions.

It is important to make note of other health care professionals—physicians, psychologists, chiropractors, body-oriented therapists—that are working with the client. For ethical and legal purposes, you should assure and document that the client is receiving adequate medical care. If the client is, in your opinion, not adequately served, then referrals and strong recommendations should be made and documented since Healing Touch is a complementary approach. Another reason for determining the client's other professionals is for networking and developing understanding of your work in the community.

Listen to what the client's body is telling you. The body is a perfect feedback system if we allow ourselves to pay attention. From the holistic perspective, discomfort and malfunction are signals that something further is needed for wholeness. Although traditional medical approaches may be to cut out or remove the broken part, the energetic view is to learn from the symptoms. Pain, for example, is a useful signal, much like a fire alarm. If we simply eliminate the pain with medication, we get a temporary solution, like taking the batteries out of the fire alarm. In the long run this removal of symptoms does not help us to deal with the underlying problem. However, if we ask when, how often, and under what circumstances the pain occurs, we can learn how to prevent its onset or minimize the distress. We might ask, then, not so much *what* the specific problems are but rather *which* client, with certain energetic and stress patterns, has this particular problem.

***Assessment***   Assessment of the energy field with the hands is like an interview, only one done with the hands. Our bodies are symmetrical and should feel the same on both sides. In wellness, the energy flows evenly from head to toe without blocks, breaks, unevenness, or temperature variations. Any disruption of the flow reflects disharmony in that area and suggests the need for further exploration.

Approach the client from a centered state, releasing any preconceived notions about what you might find. Determine the shape of the energy field by slowly scanning its outer edges. Start 3 to 4 feet away from the body and move toward it using the palms as sensors. Continue until you can determine the actual outline of the energy field.

The ways that energy is sensed in the field include temperature differentials, ridges over painful areas, blockage of energy flow, disorganized patterns, "pulls," or protective armoring. Pain may feel like needles, prickly, buzzing, or shooting darts. Blocks may feel still, sluggish, heavy, hollow, sticky, or compacted. Disorganized energy feels rough, bumpy, static, or ruffled with whorls of erratic flows. "Pulls" feel like depletion, emptiness, sucking, grasping, or pushing. Protective armoring has very definite boundaries and serves to encapsulate or protect a vulnerable area.

The healer continues the assessment by feeling the vital layer of the field, 1 to 6 inches off the skin, and by moving toward the body. The chakras in the palms of the hands are the receptors that pick up differences in temperature and pressure and other information. These receptors sense warmth and coolness that is quite different from the physical temperature of the hand, which you can test by placing your hand on the client's skin.

As you sense the energy field, you are usually aware of temperature differences first, and then you begin to notice pulsation, vibrations, or turbulence. Remember to be very alert, as changes are subtle and may happen quickly even as you are assessing. You want to be able to identify areas in relation to the physical body where the field is different, perhaps not as vibrant or as smooth as in other areas.

Note also the energy of each chakra or center as described in chapter 6. Each chakra has its own unique vibrational pattern and will feel different from the field as a whole. With experience, you will be able to detect the chakras as you move your hands over the vortices since the sensation feels like something is brushing your hand. Comparison can be made between the centers so that you can determine which ones are open and which ones are blocked and unable to receive the flow from the Universal Energy Field.

***Documentation*** Documentation of the assessment begins with the initial client contact and continues throughout the entire visit. Mentally make note of all sensations, even the ones that may seem very subtle. You may need to devise your own vocabulary for these subtle perceptions, such as "full," "empty," "dense," because of the subjective nature of the observations. A picture of the energy pattern is usually easy to do by drawing the perceived pattern on a simple outline of the body. Areas of energetic differences can be drawn in as can injuries, swelling, scars, or the track of a pain ridge. Colors can be added to denote areas where you sensed color, especially in relation to the chakras. Brightness or dullness are other ways that we visually distinguish the differences between blocked and open centers.

***Intervention*** The practitioner can choose many healing interventions in the sequence, such as the ones described in chapters 9 to 11. The art of healing comes in being able to make intelligent choices for the greatest effectiveness. The more the healer can learn about the various energetic modalities, the wiser the choice. During the intervention time, which may last 20 to 30 minutes, all of the healer's skill and prior experience is utilized. Thus, knowledge of counseling or of issues the client might encounter when in an altered state of consciousness add further depth to the healing work.

***Completion and Grounding*** After completion of the interventions, carefully ground the client. One way to do this is to hold the feet until you sense a flow and connection with the client and sense that the client's energy is back in the feet. Another way is to brush down the body from head to toe and down the arms toward the ground. Do this briskly several times. Often, clients will spontaneously start moving their hands and feet as they reconnect fully with the body. You may also choose to give a suggestion, "Feel your fingers, and your toes; now gently move them until you return to full awareness in this room."

After suggesting a return to awareness in the present, spend some time with the client to obtain feedback. Focus on what the client experienced, helping him to stay with the immediacy of the moment. Note what you sensed as the client describes his process. Talking helps the client to feel grounded as well. Carefully determine that the client is fully alert before allowing him to leave. It is also useful to reassess the energy field at this time and to document the changes.

*Follow-up Visits*   One healing sequence is sometimes adequate for clients to achieve their goals, but frequently more than one session is indicated. For long-term or chronic problems, considerable repatterning of the energy field is needed on a weekly basis. If the person has acute symptoms, more frequent visits may be necessary to help hold the energy field open. Teaching the client's family members or friends specific interventions that you found most helpful is a good way to enhance the time between visits. If medical treatment is also being given, make sure you get laboratory findings and test reports to monitor progress. Also, be aware of the need to adjust medications if side effects develop. Overall, let the client's responses to your energetic interventions determine the rate of progress, and set a schedule that seems logical to you.

*Completion of the Work*   Discharge planning begins with the initial visit as the goals of the healing work are set. The end objective is to find the optimum choices for the client and to have the resource people available for this through referrals. Although complete well-being is our hope, this may not be possible within our human time frame. Sometimes there is an obvious need for surgical intervention, and the healer can assist by preparing the client and offering support throughout the surgical process. At other times, the need for psychotherapy is evident, and the healer would refer unless she is also a qualified therapist.

If the client is no longer in need of energetic intervention but wishes to maintain the contact for prevention and health enhancement, a more relaxed schedule can evolve. In such a case, the client determines the pacing of visits unless there is a change in the client's condition that requires more frequent visits.

# THE HEALING TOUCH PRACTITIONER

Most practitioners of energy-based therapies begin with a basic education in a health care profession like nursing, counseling, or massage. Depending on their state's licensing laws related to touching clients for a fee, they can add the specific training in Healing Touch to their credentials and proceed to practice. Non-health professionals can work privately within the family setting, assisting others as a first aid intervention, as part of a healing ministry, and for self-care, always within the scope of adequate medical care. If nonprofessionals wish to do Healing Touch in a more public way, they need to obtain the appropriate education and licensure required in their state.

Persons taking Healing Touch courses can become certified through Healing Touch International, Inc. Certification is a national recognition of persons who have attended and integrated the carefully sequenced educational and mentorship process to become Certified Healing Touch Practitioners (CHTP). The criteria for certification of Healing Touch Practitioners are listed in Appendix B. Our experience shows that it usually takes two to three years for very mature and committed individuals to complete the training program and become ready for certification.

The Healing Touch training program is recognized as a continuing education program for nurses through the American Nurses Credentialing Center's Commission on Accreditation (ANCC) and is endorsed by the American Holistic Nurses' Association (AHNA). The program is also recognized as a continuing education program for massage therapists through the National Certification Board for Therapeutic Massage and Bodywork (NCBTMB).

The true significance of certification as a recognition of energy-based practitioners rests in the future, as it has only been in effect since 1994. Much will depend on the insight, skill, and wisdom that the Healing Touch practitioners demonstrate and their ability to communicate effectively with others. Ultimately, the consumer who experiences our work will determine its value and seek out effective caregivers.

## SUMMARY

We see now how the careful preparation of the practitioner becomes the foundation of a dynamic, integrated practice. As we have stated, balancing of the energy field is a necessary complement to other modalities, like psychotherapy, massage, body-oriented approaches, and traditional medical practice. We might think of energy work as the missing piece in the current health care picture. We will explore these vital linkages with other disciplines in the next section.

# Healing Touch Practice as a Complement to Other Healing Modalities

*As we have suggested throughout the book, Healing Touch is a modality that best serves as a complement or an adjunct to other modalities. In the next three chapters we will explore the ways in which this energetic work enhances and interfaces with the traditional practices of medicine, somatic therapies, and psychotherapy.*

# CHAPTER 13

# Bridges with Medical and Clinical Settings

> *"Local theories of the mind are not only incomplete, they are destructive. They create the illusion of death and aloneness, altogether local concepts. They foster existential oppression and hopelessness by giving us an utterly false idea of our basic nature. . . . This local scenario is ghastly, and it is regrettable that it continues to dominate the picture put forth by most of our best psychologists and bioscientists."*
>
> —L. Dossey., 1989

## INTRODUCTION

As the above quote suggests, the medical profession and its related helping professionals have defined their domains too narrowly. By focusing predominantly on the physical realm, opportunities for healing in other arenas are missed. Many patients and families feel abandoned by their medical practitioners just when they most need assistance, as in experiencing severe, debilitating diseases, chronic pain, or terminal illness.

Larry Dossey, MD, is an internist with many years of experience who writes about ways this misplaced concreteness severely limits and constricts the work of health care professionals (Dossey, 1997; 1998; 1999). Over and over in medical practice one meets the exceptional patient who improves despite the worst prognosis. There are also the many who expire when they have given up hope. In constricting understanding to a local view—the mind as contained in the physical brain—many physicians also see death as the ultimate end and, therefore, as failure. When we can begin to see consciousness as infinite, in a nonlocal way, then moral, ethical, and spiritual considerations become more important. Physicians may, for example, begin to talk about the quality of life that a certain technology can give rather than unquestioningly utilizing life-prolonging measures. Or they might consider the ways in which the patient can heal emotionally and spiritually to have a positive and conscious death.

# TOWARD AN INTEGRATIVE MEDICINE

Other physicians and thinkers are writing about more expanded views of the mind as well. A family practitioner who works with Native American populations in the Southwest, Dr. Hammerschlag, has found that physicians are seen as empowered beings, like the priests of the past, who can help persuade the individual to heal. "If belief helps a patient to find comfort, and if we believe we can help patients, then we must invoke the power of all healing sacraments to do so— to help the patient grow and heal, or even to accept losses and death" (Hammerschlag, 1989, p. 87). In learning to become a healer, he found that patients do not need a scientist who knows facts but rather a caring person who helps them to find connections between themselves and their inner being, and between themselves and the transpersonal dimensions.

In a more scientific vein, Richard Gerber, MD, addresses the basis for a new paradigm of medical practice in *Vibrational Medicine* (1988; 1996; 2001). The shift in science from the atomic, fragmented Newtonian worldview to the unbroken wholeness of Einstein and the quantum mechanical worldview is gradually impacting every part of our lives. This includes how we see the body, its relation to mind, and the universe in which we live. Gerber's works elaborate in detail how healing, via systems that affect the subtle energies, is an extension of existing medical science just as the Einsteinian viewpoint is an extension of the Newtonian physics. If all matter is really energy, as Einstein insists, then we must see the human body as a dynamic, interactive energy system and develop ways to work with this energy for healing.

Whether individual bioscientists and medical practitioners believe this new model of the world or not is relatively unimportant. The fact is that science is progressing rapidly beyond our wildest fantasies. The effectiveness of existing medical technology is constantly enhanced by new, adjunctive discoveries. MRI (magnetic resonance imaging), for example, is energetic in principle. The atoms under study, usually hydrogen, are stimulated by the transfer of energy at a specific frequency. The energy is only absorbed by the atom if it is of a particular resonant frequency such as that of healthy cells. Thus, an energetic picture of the area to be studied unfolds giving the analyst images of healthy or defective structures in the tissues (Gerber, 2001, pp. 104–106).

Other research in the field of neurotransmitters and neuropeptides points to the complex interactions of the body and mind. It is no longer enough to look at the isolated parts of neuroanatomy because the whole is apparently much more than the sum of its parts. Although the hard sciences have largely ignored consciousness and intuition, the physical body is now understood to be exquisitely connected to thought and emotions. The body matches our thought patterns instantly through the biochemical changes within the neuropeptides and their receptors (Pert, 1997) and we can accurately speak of *bodymind* as one integrated concept.

Another sign of change within medical thinking is the tremendous public response that Deepak Chopra, MD, has received in speaking about Ayurvedic medicine based on age-old Eastern Indian traditions. In a time of highly developed medical technologies, Chopra found his spirit hungry despite high achievements as an endocrinologist and as chief of staff at a New England hospital. He turned to learning from the inner wisdom of the body, "the organizing power that flows from its deep source in the self and coordinates every aspect of the physical system" (1991, p. 202). Meditation became his vehicle for accessing this inner wisdom. Meditation or centering focuses the mind, but it also permits activation of the parasympathetic nervous system's responses and the biochemical changes that produce endorphins and increase functioning of the immune system (Chopra, 1997; Anand & Chopra, 2000).

## Complementary Practices

The times seem ripe for numerous complementary approaches to augment the tremendous strides that have been made in the biochemical sciences. These complementary practices can enhance medical practice by incorporating the energetic model of quantum physics, the bodymind understanding of psychoneuroimmunology, and the holistic view of interacting systems that are much more than their individual parts. As pioneer physician Dr. Benor emphasizes, complementary practice that includes energy healing concepts is the medicine of the future (Benor, 2001).

# HEALING TOUCH AS A COMPLEMENTARY APPROACH

Healing Touch can rightly be seen as one of these complementary approaches. As the following examples show, there are many applications for hospital and clinical settings that allow the patient to receive the best possible care, not only physically but emotionally, and at more subtle energetic levels. Thus, Healing Touch can extend the medical practitioner's treatment plan to include aspects that could not be addressed by traditional means. Finding ways that the client can extend his self-care and become an active participant in improving health (Coleman & Gurin, 1993) is an essential component of modern medical care. Healing Touch offers excellent resources for such self-care and thus becomes a viable adjunct to personal health maintenance.

## Pre- and Postprocedural Care

Many medical procedures, including surgery, chemotherapy, and complex diagnostic testing, produce anxiety in the client, even prior to their onset. A simple Healing Touch technique like the Magnetic Unruffle done 5 minutes before the procedure can help the client to feel less distraught and remind him of his internal resources for coping with stress. An energy field technique combined with relaxation imagery can be even more powerful so that preoperative medication can be kept to a minimum.

In the time after a medical procedure, smoothing of the energy field, especially at the intervention site, is necessary. Assessment of the field by hand scan or penduling often shows that the area is depleted, flat, or cold in spite of the fact that a wound is physically sealed. This suggests that something further is needed to rebalance the energy flows, otherwise the client may report feeling "drained" or "fragmented" even months later.

Several Healing Touch students on the West Coast are dermatological surgeons who excise facial tumors on a daily basis. They have found unruffling the energy field a helpful way to start preoperative preparation. They find that the patient needs less local anesthesia and is more relaxed during the operation. At the end, these caring surgeons put their energy into the wound dressing and smooth the entire field before the patient leaves. Stitches can often be removed earlier than the usual 7 days because of accelerated wound healing when Healing Touch is used.

Because of advances of medical science, many persons are alive with severe illnesses that require repeated treatments. Kidney dialysis, for example, is repeated three times a week and can prolong life for many years until a suitable transplant is found. In spite of the wonders of this technology, many dialysis patients undergo severe personal and emotional stresses related to the procedures that make their daily life almost unbearable. The human toll in anxiety is something that

## JOAN'S STORY

Recently, I worked with a young dialysis patient named Joan, whose presenting problem was a severe needle phobia that made the frequent trips to the dialysis center an unimaginable ordeal. No amount of medication or tranquilizing agent made an impact. Bit by bit, I taught Joan how to use the Ultrasound technique over the needle insertion sites along with an affirmation, a repeated positive statement, to comfort her inner fears. To this we added creative imaging of peaceful scenes and pictures of the goals for which she was staying alive. Her practice was so successful that the shunt lasted for more than 5 years, a time sufficient to prepare for a transplant. Even though the implant operation was to take place many miles from home, Joan felt quite relaxed because, through our networks, the Healing Touch nurses from that community came to assist her before and after surgery.

medical science has few means to address. However, preprocedural fears can be diminished with Healing Touch and some of the self-care techniques suggested in chapter 17. The disarray of the person's energy field after dialysis responds well to energetic rebalancing by a family member.

## Assisting with Incurable Illness

Many medical practices deal with severe, physically incurable illnesses such as cancer and AIDS. Again, it makes sense to look for other ways to assist the patient when medical science has reached its limits. "There is nothing further we can do for you" is a verdict that not only creates a feeling of hopelessness in the sufferer, but also denies the existence of many other resources (Eliopoulos, 1999).

Several publications speak of the personality profiles of exceptional cancer patients with stage IV, widely metastatic disease. "The patients who significantly outlived their expectancy were more creative, more receptive to new ideas, flexible and argumentative. They had strong egos and expressed feelings of personal adequacy and vitality. . . . They sought out innovative medical treatment, refusing to accept the death sentence handed out with their diagnosis. In this sense, they were seen as using a form of denial—not denying the seriousness of their disease by any means, but denying that they would be victims" (Achterberg, 1985, p. 180).

The vitalizing techniques of HT that work from the lower body to the higher levels give many options for persons with severe and debilitating conditions. In

## JIM'S STORY

Jim was a singer and dancer whose love of life bubbled over into every aspect of his AIDS diagnosis. He was unwilling to accept the medical facts by preparing for death. Instead, he wanted to learn ways of making the best possible use of the time he had.

Despite deep bouts of depression, he began to create pictures and songs out of his pain. He used the Chakra Connection on himself daily and whenever he felt tired or "out of kilter." His wife noticed how, despite his neuropathy, his mind stayed alert with the Mind Clearing technique through the pain and physical chaos. Most importantly, Jim no longer felt powerless; he had ways of dealing with difficult times.

Jim long outlived his life expectancy, learning about his humanness and about his connections with Higher Power. "Every day is a gift," he said. "The songs and melodies just keep coming. I hope my songs will help someone else to see their light."

addition, there are many techniques that the family can learn to assist the individual, such as the Magnetic Unruffle and the Chakra Connection. And, the client can feel empowered himself by centering and modifying techniques to be self-help resources, for example Ultrasound and Pain Drain. If the client chooses to live consciously, every day can be filled with meaning and purpose despite the limitations of the physical body.

## Supporting Healing while Someone is Dying

Although the idea of healing through the experience of dying may sound paradoxical, our expanded holistic view of healing suggests that every moment of life has potential for healing. Where the physical body is unable to recover, other aspects of the biofield may become activated and unexpected moments of grace emerge. I learned this very directly when I was called to assist with a terminally ill two-year old. The healing that occurred for the family was beyond my wildest expectations and I will always be grateful for the gifts of that day. My only resources were to be fully centered throughout the experience and to provide simple smoothing of the child's biofield along with one round of the Chakra Spread.

### LITTLE PAUL'S STORY

A call came from a businessman who had read about little Paul in the newspaper. The two-and-a-half-year-old boy desperately needed a bone marrow transplant for severe leukemia, but by the time the businessman had raised the money, the child was too ill for surgery. In desperation, the gentleman called me, having heard about Healing Touch through a friend. He wanted me to visit the family and fix everything. I attempted to explain about the complementary nature of energy-based work and that physical healing might not be the result of my visit. Undeterred, he insisted that I go to the family and share what I knew.

Although I agreed, I felt my resistance to the project. Why should I go, perhaps to help the child die? Then I remembered that often the various techniques of Healing Touch could be a resource when traditional medical practice, especially as we know it in the West, had reached the end of its capabilities. Steeled with this thought, I called the parents, who expressed great eagerness to meet with me.

A warm greeting from both parents assured me that I was not intruding. They were eager to learn about energy, and I shared some pictures of the human energy field. When I saw little Paul, I recognized the face of impending death. His skin was ash-colored, his little eyes opened and rolled back in his head, and his breathing was labored and erratic. I

*(continues)*

*Little Paul's Story (continued)*

recalled that energy-related therapy often facilitates easy transition to dimensions beyond this life. I felt there was a real possibility that Paul might pass on as I did Healing Touch with him.

Shoring up all the resources I could muster, I spoke with the parents about healing in other dimensions. If the physical could not improve, we might see a balancing in the emotions, increased mental clarity, or direct connecting with the spiritual/intuitive dimensions. They understood my meaning and asked me to help in any way I could. "You see, the doctors gave up on Paul over a week ago. We feel abandoned since they said there is nothing further they could do. We are obviously in need and Paul is still alive. Please stay with us awhile."

My heart reached out to them and their dilemma. As the father and mother took turns holding the frail body, I began smoothing the child's biofield. Whenever I came closer than two feet, Paul would whine a little and brush me away, so I knew the boundaries of his energy field and continued the motion at a distance. I followed with the chakra spread and a gentle modulation energy above the heart center. I also taught the parents how to balance their own heart centers to increase relaxation and immune system functioning.

Fully expecting Paul to sleep or pass on, I was amazed when he clearly said, "I want milk" after about twenty minutes. His eyes became more alert, and, after finishing his milk, he wanted to go for a bike ride. When I left, Paul was sitting upright on his own in his little chair waiting to go for a ride with his dad. I looked into his eyes and saw the clear gaze of eternity looking back at me.

The next day was Good Friday, and I dreamed that Paul had left his physical body. The Monday after Easter his father called to tell me that Paul had, indeed, died on Good Friday but not until he had played with the family for three hours, and everyone, even relatives, had been able to say farewell. "That Thursday afternoon was the greatest gift we could ever have received," his father said. "It was just like old times: we played and laughed and ate and slept soundly that night. The next morning both my wife and I told Paul that we would understand if he needed to go on. We were ready to release him, and in twelve hours he was gone."

# Helping with Birthing and Neonates

Just as the energy-related work assists those exiting, so it is relevant in helping people coming into life. Krieger's studies with families before the birth of their child show that tremendous bonding that can happen as the couple prepares by sensing the child's and the family's energy field (Krieger, 1993, pp. 138–143).

One of our practitioners is a nurse midwife we'll call Ruth. She has her own private practice and also regularly assists with births at a local hospital. From the beginning of labor until several hours after the birth, she fosters relaxation in the mothers by doing the Magnetic Unruffle and the Chakra Spread. Smoothing the baby's energy field after birth with a few short sweeps calms the little one and often brings a wide-eyed smile.

Ruth has also found Healing Touch techniques very helpful with neonates, especially those that are having physical difficulties. Since medication is usually contraindicated, she uses unruffling over the area or Ultrasound for reaching deep into the tissues.

Particularly heartrending are the cries of addicted babies who, because of the mother's drug abuse, must detoxify right after birth. Jane, another Healing Touch practitioner, found that short periods of smoothing repeated every hour yield the best results. In the children's hospital of a southwestern community, Jane is a bit of a legend because her touch, often just above the biofield, brings rapid change in these cranky and irritable babies.

# Geriatric Care

Another largely underserved population are the elderly. For simple aches and pains to severe confusion due to organic brain changes, Healing Touch can be a valuable resource. Many psychiatric units harbor large geriatric populations that often frustrate the caregivers. We have seen a dramatic impact when nurses center together at the beginning of a shift, unruffle and modulate energy with each other as needed, and design treatment plans that include Healing Touch. Although the calming of an agitated geriatric patient may only be temporary due to neurological damage, the intervention may be sufficient to accomplish a task or to establish rapport. A number of day treatment centers for the elderly are including Healing Touch in their programs and report such results as centering, calming, and a sense of personal empowerment. Some of the more responsive clients enjoy sharing Healing Touch techniques with the other participants in the program (personal communication, Joslyn Senior Center, Rancho Bernardo, CA, 2001).

# Dealing with Long-Term Pain

Although the effects of energy-related interventions for postoperative pain have been well documented, less is known about the impact of such interventions on chronic, long-term pain. Sufferers of severe pain syndrome often travel from physician to physician looking for relief. As ever-increasing doses of pain-relieving medication are prescribed, they are prone to addiction because tolerance sets in when neurotransmitters and receptor sites become blocked. The body's capacity to produce its own endorphins and enkephalins for pain relief is diminished as increasing doses of medication impact the system. All too frequently, the depression that results from years of this pain cycle leads to psychiatric disorder and admission to either a psychiatric care facility or a pain management unit.

Nothing moves quickly once the pattern of pain has been established, usually over several years, yet most persons in pain want instant relief, miracles on the double. It is important, then, to educate the pain patient that relief can at best be measured in small increments. We may talk about a 5% improvement or a shift from a subjective unit of distress of "9" discomfort to a "7". The important thing to note is that there is a slight shift with the energy therapy and to suggest that, from then on, gradual changes may develop over weeks and months. If there is no response whatever to Healing Touch techniques, it is wise to conclude that the client's energy field is not able to respond and that some other modality may be more appropriate.

It goes without saying that anyone with a severe pain problem should work closely under a physician's supervision. Our experience is that most specialists in this type of medicine are pleased to have additional resources as they as individuals are quickly exhausted by the client's ongoing demands for medication and

## PATTI'S STORY

Patti was a nurse in a hospital that combines pain management with psychiatric care. She found that pain patients disliked the unit because they felt they had different issues. Consequently, the pain patients would not participate in the community activities on the unit, and their participation in therapy groups was lackluster at best. Clearly, something else was needed. So Patti quietly began unruffling the painful areas of the patients who were open to the idea. She later taught them HT self-help techniques as well as relaxation skills.

Participation at the evening meetings to relax before bedtime reached an all-time high when the pain patients were joined by psychiatric patients. All of them found they could sleep better after Patti's sessions than with medication alone. The patients were also more receptive and available for psychotherapy the next morning.

The patients began telling their physicians about their experiences. The physicians became curious, and, when they understood what Patti was doing, they wrote a standing order for HT to be used prn (as needed), at the nurse's discretion.

comforting. Currently, a number of Healing Touch practitioners are working successfully in conjunction with pain management clinics.

## DOCUMENTATION

As with all practices that may seem novel or innovative to the inexperienced, careful documentation of Healing Touch is essential. First, the Healing Touch practitioner must always insure that the client is receiving adequate medical care by carefully asking and documenting information about recent medical history and physical examinations. If the client refuses traditional medical care, physicians who practice integrative medicine may be consulted. Fortunately, through computerized networks, few patients are limited to local practitioners since most have access to a vast array of national resources.

Next, the Healing Touch practitioner needs to document his assessment of the biofield and chakras, the energetic patterns that, in addition to identification of physical and emotional issues, become the foundation of the nursing, or other practitioner, diagnosis. This diagnosis then becomes the foundation of a purposeful plan of care that may include Healing Touch interventions and referral to other resources. This intentional planning can be carried out in hospital settings in a few minutes or take place over several weeks and months in out-patient settings, as those described by Janet Mentgen in chapter 12.

Careful documentation of the interventions that are used and their effects, both immediate and over time, gives the practitioner feedback and further directs the plan of care. For example, a nurse may find that pain medication coupled with the Magnetic Unruffle allows pain relief more quickly in a certain patient. Documentation and reporting of these effects will allow other shifts to use a similar approach and to learn more about effects of working with energy healing. Communication with colleagues, other professionals, and even family members is essential as we think of the vast network of interactive human energy fields and the environment of caring that can be generated.

## SUMMARY

We can certainly say that Healing Touch has high relevance as a complement to medical care. There are probably as many applications of this work as the individual practitioner's interest and creativity allow. The work can be integrated unobtrusively in most health care settings and is often initiated by the consumer's request.

When approaching physicians, it is important to communicate clearly the research and scientific base and to be sensitive to the possibility of fear or caution on the part of traditional practitioners. Ultimately, it is the feedback from the client that is most valuable in showing how Healing Touch enhances medical out-comes. Hence, good documentation of the initial assessment, interventions used, and evaluation of the client after each intervention is essential.

# REFERENCES

Achterberg, J. (1985). *Imagery and healing*. Boston: New Science Library, Shambala.

Anand, M. & Chopra, D. (2000). *The art of everyday ecstasy*. Audiotape. LaJolla, CA: Chopra Center for Well-Being.

Benor, D. J. (2001). *Spiritual healing*. Vol I–IV. (Rev. ed.) Southfield, MI: Vision Publications.

Chopra, D. (1991). *Return of the rishi*. Boston: Houghton-Mifflin Co.

Chopra, D. (1997). *Boundless energy: the complete mind/body program for overcoming chronic fatigue*. New York: Perfect Health Library Series, No. 3.

Coleman, D., & Gurin, J. (1993). *Mindbody medicine*. Yonkers, NY: Consumer Reports Books.

Dossey, L. (1989). *Recovering the soul* (p. 7). New York: Bantam Books.

Dossey, L. (1997). *Healing words*. San Francisco, CA: Harper Collins.

Dossey, L. (1998). *Be careful what you pray for. . .you just might get it*. San Francisco, CA: Harper Collins.

Dossey, L. (1999). *Reinventing medicine*. San Francisco, CA: Harper Collins.

Eliopoulos, C. (1999). *Integrating conventional and alternative therapies: Holistic care for chronic conditions*. St. Louis, MO: C. V. Mosby Co.

Gerber, R. (1988; 1996; 2001). *Vibrational medicine*. Rochester, VT: Bear and Co.

Hammerschlag, C. (1989). *The dancing healers*. San Francisco: HarperCollins Publishers.

Krieger, D. (1993). *Accepting your power to heal*. Santa Fe, NM: Bear and Co.

Pert, C. (1997). *Molecules of emotion*. New York: Charles Scribner's Sons.

# CHAPTER 14

# Interfaces with Somatic Therapies

*"Energy is the real substance behind the appearance of matter and form."*

—R. Stone quoted in Chitty & Muller, 1990

## INTRODUCTION

This quote from the founder of Polarity Therapy reminds us of the many ways that energy-based concepts currently interface with body-oriented, somatic therapies. In fact, one of the most asked questions in our Healing Touch (HT) classes is how HT is related to or different from somatic approaches such as massage, Reiki, or polarity.

In this chapter we will explore some of the ways that HT can be utilized readily by somatic therapists. HT can be integrated into the body worker's specialty practice because of its broad and basic approach to the human energy system. HT differs from the many body-related therapies in that the practice of HT requires less specific anatomical knowledge and includes awareness of the dimensions of the biofield and chakras.

## BODY-RELATED THERAPIES

In the past 30 years especially, there has been increasing interest in ways to maintain optimum functioning and wellness in the physical body. The general public began asking questions about rising health care costs and means of preventing physical problems. Since medical science has largely focused on the diagnosis and treatment of disease, many individuals began turning to alternatives for health maintenance and self-improvement even without the consultation or approval of their physicians (Eisenberg et al., 1998). Those who chose alternative means of staying well began exploring the wide and growing field of somatic therapies. Many of these alternative approaches define health as a function of subtle energy that flows within the body and is obstructed or congested in illness. Thus, increasing self-awareness among the public has fostered insight about energy and intuition. Beyond physical exercise, the more adventurous seekers learned breathing and movement for relaxation and stress reduction and received various forms of touch therapies to soothe the body (Anselmo & Kolkmeier, 2000).

Body-related therapies, then, are often the layperson's first exposure to a more integrated view of the bodymind and the idea of doing more to maintain health than merely consulting one's physician. Massage, for example, has renewed its time-honored place as the art and science of muscle relaxation through specific, skillful manipulation of muscle tissue (Lidell, 1984; Mitzel-Wilkinson, 2000). To assure a professional status for massage, most states require a specified number of educational hours and identified skills to license the practitioner to administer touch. Advanced training for massage therapists has led to development and certification of a wide variety of related specialty techniques—reflexology, polarity therapy, Shiatzu, and Feldenkrais, to name a few.

A wide variety of touch approaches and techniques are included under the broad heading of somatic, or body-oriented therapies. Except for the energy modalities, like HT and Therapeutic Touch, all body therapies include actual physical contact. "The contact usually consists of the practitioner's touching, pushing, kneading, or rubbing the recipient's skin and underlying fascia tissue. Each of the therapies has its own body of knowledge, history, and technique" (Shames & Keegan, 2000).

# HEALING TOUCH AS A COMPLEMENT TO SOMATIC THERAPIES

## Massage

HT is an excellent complement to massage therapy, especially when pain or open sores make usual deep tissue work inappropriate. It is also useful as an opening in a massage session to help prepare the client and establish rapport with the client's energy field. Another option is to use HT techniques at the end of a massage treatment to bring the layers of the biofield into balance.

June, a licensed massage therapist, found that HT interventions allowed her to work at much deeper levels with her clients. She discovered, for example, that dense muscle tissue often separates more easily when the client is in the relaxed state that is available quickly through HT. June's clients often responded more quickly to her work with the biofield. June likens her blending of the two approaches to an etheric massage in which all layers of the field, not just the physical, are included.

HT practice does not require the specific anatomical knowledge of massage work, although it is useful for the practitioner to have this information. To differentiate from massage, HT works either with a light touch on the body or moving the hands in the biofield above the body. Also, no draping or disrobing is required for the client to receive Healing Touch as the emphasis is on working with clients wherever they are, whether in the emergency room, in a hospital bed, in a private office, or in a home setting.

There is a wealth of information to be shared as talented body workers incorporate HT into their practices. Many clients are highly sensitive and ready for multilevel work because of their personal seeking for higher levels of wellness. The following stories are examples of the interchanges of skilled body workers and sensitive, attuned clients who were able to benefit fully from the added dimension of energetic interventions.

## DONNA'S STORY

A massage client we'll call Donna complained of a lifelong problem with "tired feet." No matter what the expense, no shoes ever fit or felt right to her. As June, the masseuse, began unruffling the biofield, Donna reported increasing discomfort and tingly sensations in her feet that she had not previously experienced. As the pain increased, June slowed her movements, moved further out into the biofield, and gently held her focus, sending caring thoughts to Donna's entire being. Suddenly, Donna experienced an emotional and physical release, almost like an auditory pop, as the field cleared spontaneously. June completed the session by gently smoothing the problem areas and making sure Donna was fully alert before leaving the office. Since that time, Donna has had no further discomfort with her shoes and experiences living fully in her body, including her feet.

## CAROL'S STORY

Carol was a fascinating client. As a psychic consultant she was able to help many people, but her own sense of imbalance in the physical body persisted. As her massage therapist, Joe, assessed her energy field, he found marked lateral imbalance. The right and left sides of her body and even her face looked different. She described herself as "not quite together." Joe dropped his usual massage routine explaining he would work to help rebalance her field. As he proceeded with the Magnetic Unruffle, Carol felt a weaving pattern across the middle of her body, almost as if the

*(continues)*

*Carol's Story (continued)*

two halves were being rejoined. Since she was highly intuitive, she saw colors ranging from yellow to blue as Joe worked, and she felt gentle releasing, like feathers brushing against the skin of her neck. Since that session, she has felt "together," lost 20 pounds, and no longer seeks traditional massage. Instead, Carol goes for monthly rebalancing of her biofield as Joe continues to learn about the colors of the human energy system from his interactions with her.

## Blending with Reiki

Reiki is an ancient Sanskrit tradition that is currently growing in popularity (Lidell, 1984). Reiki is described by a practitioner as an adjunctive therapy for relaxation and pain relief in which "…Practitioners gently rest their hands in specific ways on approximately 12 standard sites throughout the body, which may vary slightly among practitioners. Reiki practitioners begin with the head and spend a few minutes at each site, with a complete session taking 60-90 minutes" (O' Mathuna, 1999). Like Healing Touch, Reiki is based on the belief that all life depends on a universal, nonphysical energy that needs to be balanced within the individual for optimum functioning.

In contrast, HT allows much more flexibility. As noted, some of the specific interventions listed in chapters 9 to 11 can be done in 5 minutes, and allow the healer the option of returning at a later time to do more. There is also movement with HT that permits the healer to find a problem site and to work over the most congested areas, then later to complete the work with modulation of energy or hand holds. So, again, the combination of the two modalities would allow for optimum results through a skilled practitioner.

## Integration with Deep Tissue Work

A number of somatic therapies work deep in the tissues or cause actual movement of bone. Among these we can list neuromuscular and trigger point therapies as well as craniosacral manipulation (Upledger, 1997). As we might expect, these approaches require careful training in anatomy and affect primarily the physical aspect of the energy field. The possibility of harm is a concern as each person's body may respond differently to external pressure and manipulation. In contrast, HT does not require any pressure or manipulation because trust is placed in the inner wisdom of the body and the field to respond to the gentle energy interventions in whatever way is needed.

In energy-based therapy we learn that muscles can relax one by one, sometimes over several sessions. As muscles lengthen and tension is released, bone sutures and small joints naturally realign themselves, often reversing the sequence of the injury pathway. In addition, the client has an opportunity to learn to listen to the body and note how each movement augments or diminishes relaxation.

## Communication with Polarity Therapists

Polarity therapy is another form of body therapy that is currently popular. Many of the concepts taught in polarity closely resemble HT and sometimes confuse the practitioner who attempts to do both. For example, sensing energy flows with the hands is carefully taught in polarity therapy but with emphasis on direction of the *Qi* from the negative charge to the positive, the right hand to the left hand, and so forth (Sills, 1989). HT is much more spontaneous and intuitive, emphasizing the practitioner's response to the client's imbalanced *Qi*. Persons who enjoy complex cognitive learning find polarity therapy enjoyable, and the two disciplines have much to offer each other in dialogue and mutual understanding. Underlying both practices is the vision that health is a function of subtle energy flows that can be brought into balance.

## JACKIE'S STORY

To demonstrate how complex treatment of the multidimensional human being can be, we offer the case example of a 30-year-old nurse we'll call Jackie. She attended a Healing Touch class several years ago, perhaps sensing that she would need more help. Her job in the intensive care unit of a midwestern hospital was highly stressful. Two weeks after taking the class, she woke up literally unable to move or to go to work. She refused medical help and had a friend bring her to a local nurse healer. The noninvasive nature of Healing Touch relaxed her enough that she could walk with care and be seen by one of the neurologists the HT practitioner recommended. X rays showed a herniated neck disc that would require 3 months of bed rest and close observation but no surgery, according to several medical specialists. Healing Touch then became Jackie's weekly link to a whole new world of learning about her body and her emotions.

Progress seemed terribly slow to this young woman who had been used to making quick decisions and getting things done. Her compulsive nature expressed itself in housecleaning that would strain the body and send her into acute muscle spasms. This pattern repeated itself many times until depression set in. Jackie realized that a change in lifestyle had to come from within, but she continued to struggle with doing things in her old, set ways. The Healing Touch practitioner now became the patient's advocate: a link to a suitable psychiatrist to deal with the depression, a contact with

*(continues)*

*Jackie's Story (continued)*

the mental health counselor so that the energy field sessions could support the psychotherapy, the connector to the social worker who handled the workers' compensation aspect of the case, the liaison for ongoing dialogue with the neurologist, and the referral to massage therapy and Feldenkrais for facilitating muscle release.

It took more than a year before Jackie was ready to seek a new job. However, she describes the difficult year as the most incredible learning experience of her life. The Healing Touch practitioner challenged her to integrate her learnings from psychotherapy, the somatic work, and the physicians. Jackie's specific problem of shoulder outlet syndrome required a sophisticated, multidisciplinary approach. Jackie now maintains body tone with moderate aerobic exercise, and successfully holds a more relaxed job as a rehabilitation nurse. Her own experiences in healing of the *psyche* and *soma* have become translated into an asset for helping others.

## SUMMARY

In this and many similar case examples, we see how all dimensions of the biofield are involved when clients seek relief from their many tensions and old patterns. It is apparent how crucial medical and somatic therapies are to enhancing daily functioning. The client benefits further when both medical practitioners and somatic therapists include the adjunctive care of HT.

It remains now for us to explore the interface of energetic interventions in the outer dimensions of the energy field—the emotional, mental, and spiritual layers. As these domains are traditionally addressed by psychotherapists, we will explore the counseling applications of HT in the next chapter.

## REFERENCES

Anselmo, J. & Kolkmeier, L. G. (2000). In Dossey, B. et al. (Eds.), *Holistic nursing*, 3rd Edition, Gaithersburg, MD: Aspen Publishers, Inc.

Chitty, J., & Muller, M. L. (1990). *Energy exercises* (p. 5). Murietta, CA: Murietta Foundation.

Eisenberg, D. M., Davis, R. B., Ettner, S. L., Appel, S., Wilkey, S., Van Rompay, M. & Kessler, R. (1998). Trends in alternative medicine use in the United States, 1990–1997: Results of a follow-up national survey. *The Journal of the American Medical Association, 280 (18), 1569–1575.*

Lidell, L. (1984). *The book of massage*. New York: Simon and Schuster.

Mitzel-Wilkinson, A. (Jan., 2000). Massage therapy as a nursing practice. *Holistic Nursing Practice, 14* (2), 48–56.

O'Mathuna, D. P. (1999). Reiki as an adjunctive therapy for relaxation and pain relief. In *Alternative Medicine Alert, 2* (12), 136. Atlanta, GA: American Health Consultants.

Shames, K. H. & Keegan, L. (2000). In Dossey, B. et al. (Eds.), *Holistic nursing,* 3rd ed., Gaithersburg, MD: Aspen.

Sills, F. (1989). *The polarity process.* Dorset, England: Selement Books.

Upledger, J. (1997). *Your inner physician and you.* Berkeley, CA: North Atlantic.

# CHAPTER 15

# Interrelationships with Psychotherapy

*"The body has memory and stores emotional experiences. At some point our inner wisdom guides us to the opportunities to release these stored memories, lest they block our energy flow and weaken our life force."*

—K. Shames, Healing Touch practitioner, personal communication, 2001

## INTRODUCTION

The numerous possibilities for direct applications of Healing Touch in the practice of psychotherapy will be explored in this chapter but first, a word about referrals. As the case of Jackie (see chapter 14) illustrated, a collaborative approach among various health care professionals can effect results that would not be possible with any single practitioner. We want to emphasize the importance of referrals to other skilled practitioners to ensure the best possible care for the client. Although it is imperative that the Healing Touch practitioner refer for medical supervision, referrals to somatic therapists with specialties beyond the techniques of energy-based work can also be very timely and helpful. Similarly, suggesting a competent psychotherapist is appropriate especially if emotional issues are surfacing and the Healing Touch practitioner does not have the expertise or qualifications to do in-depth therapy.

In our experience, referrals from other health care practitioners to the Healing Touch practitioner for energy-based work are also occurring with increasing frequency. For instance, many psychotherapists are referring clients with emotional blocks or issues that are not available for talk therapy. Energetic assessment by a Healing Touch practitioner allows the client to identify lifelong patterns in the field. As the client accesses suppressed material, blocks in the *Qi* can be released, and the client can then return to the original therapist for follow-up sessions. This kind of flexibility between health care professionals offers new options for clients and contributes significantly to resolving long-term problems more rapidly and to a greater depth than is otherwise possible.

# HEALING TOUCH AND PSYCHOTHERAPY

Many qualified psychotherapists, such as addictions specialists, marriage and family counselors, psychologists, clinical nurse specialists, and clinical social workers, have come to Healing Touch classes themselves. We want to address specific ways these counselors could utilize the concepts of Healing Touch and base our discussion on case examples they have shared. This is new material that is currently being presented to therapists at national conferences of psychological organizations like the Association of Transpersonal Psychology and the Association of Humanistic Psychology. Further sharing and mutual dialoguing is ensuing with international conferences of psychotherapists using comprehensive energy psychology. It goes without saying that the following ideas are presented as a beginning exploration of the possibilities of the new interface between psychotherapy and energy-based approaches.

## The Work of Psychotherapists

Psychotherapists with various backgrounds have an innate interest in early intervention. Whether they are aware of the layers of the energy field or not, they work with mental or emotional symptoms before they become concretized as physical problems. To put it another way, they deal with the outer layers of the biofield to prevent physical breakdown. This interest in the prevention of physical problems is manifest in the increasing literature about stress that is currently seen as the causative factor in 70–80% of physical disease (Rossi, 1986; Pert, 1997). A well-known scale actually measures in numbers the amount of distress a specific life event can cause and the likelihood of ensuing physical breakdown (Holmes & Rahe, 1967). Many of the issues that send people into psychotherapy—death of a loved one, marital discord, family strife, job-related pressures, anxiety, and experiencing a traumatic event—give opportunity for resolution at the intuitive, mental, and emotional levels of the field.

Psychotherapists also deal with the emotional and mental distress that physical illness or chemical imbalance can cause. We may think here of immune system dysfunction, such as Chronic Fatigue Syndrome, cancer, AIDS, or autoimmune disorders, as well as known chemical imbalances that cause emotional symptoms like endogenous depression and bipolar disorders. Many clients come for psychotherapy months, even years, after a medical operation that was emotionally devastating to them. To think in energetic terms, we could say the physical layer mended itself, but the emotional, mental, and/or spiritual dimensions of the biofield need further healing.

# HEALING TOUCH AS A COMPLEMENT TO PSYCHOTHERAPY

Whatever reasons clients have for seeking therapy, Healing Touch approaches offer some very effective tools to complement the eclectic skills of the caring practitioner. The full-body techniques listed in chapter 9 can be remarkably effective when paced to the individual client's needs and selected with discernment by the counselor. Rapport is established easily through light touch or smoothing the biofield, and suppressed emotions can surface quickly in a more relaxed state. Apparently, blocks in the energy field are a form of stored memory. As the therapist connects with the constricted area, the client's subconscious images, such as a repressed memory of childhood trauma, surface and can be released from the emotional layer of the field. At the same time, the therapist can assist in releasing energetic debris, and then smooth the energy layers of the chakra area to rebalance the field.

Numerous therapists have integrated Healing Touch into their practice resulting in a unique blend of energy-based concepts and counseling skills. The psychological problem areas and the condition of the energy field together give the therapist clues that can widen his resource base. In other words, the predominating emotional issue helps to determine the appropriate Healing Touch intervention that can serve as a starting place for multilevel psychotherapeutic work (Hover-Kramer & Shames, 1997).

## Comments from Psychotherapists

***Carol Lee***    Carol Lee, a clinical nurse specialist in private practice, writes:

> In my recent work, it has become apparent that I can save a lot of time and be much more connected to my client's process through monitoring the energy flow. Whereas I used to spend several sessions building trust in order that the person will eventually tell me what is affecting their health or state of "dis-ease," I am utilizing Healing Touch, with its very quick feedback mechanism, to provide energetic assessments. In our collaboration, the physician and I both notice that I am much more aware of the subtle forces operating in our clients' lives.
>
> I have also incorporated Healing Touch prior to using psychotherapy. It is my experience that the client is then more relaxed, less anxious, more present. With clients who use compulsive chatter as a means to avoid feelings, I apply the Mind Clearing techniques, which leaves them much more relaxed and present. With clients who exhibit primarily psychological disturbances, I use Healing Touch whenever they demonstrate any physical symptoms. It seems to ease the discomfort and allow for enhanced emotional release. Magentic Unruffle is very efficient in calming people down who are emotionally distraught or anxious.

***Betty*** A clinical social worker, Betty, states,

> I often use a blend of hands-on work with counseling. It seems that most people are suffering from touch deprivation rather than a lack of medication or technology in their lives. I have often witnessed the power of holding a hand or gently soothing an area of the body where there was an intense buildup of tension that the patient experienced as panic or pain in the body. In the psychiatric in-patient unit where I worked I noticed that many people could relax, sleep, or have decreased pain after a staff or family member used some form of gentle touch. Now, with the Healing Touch skills I have specific knowledge about how I can ease a client's distress and also can teach the client self-management tools.

***Jenna*** Jenna is a licensed mental health counselor who also uses massage to expand her healing capacities. She states:

> As I blended massage with psychotherapy, I witnessed some profound results. If I would touch a certain area, the patient would begin to recount an earlier experience. This made more sense to me when I understood the chakras and their functions in the Healing Touch classes. I would simply move my hands in a chakra area, even without physically touching and with the client fully clothed, encouraging the client to breathe deeply and share feelings when he felt ready to talk, and memories would just pour out.
>
> A most memorable time was when I was working with a young woman who had a dense area of heavy energy in the middle abdomen. As I unruffled with my hands in the area, she remembered having gall bladder surgery in her teens. As I touched over the area, her voice changed and she started wailing and sobbing. I continued gently moving my hands above the abdomen giving her ample time and space to express whatever she needed to get out. When the sobbing decreased, she described how her uncle had sexually abused her especially in the time before the operation. The memory of that time with all its agony and shame was imbedded in the surgical site and the related energetic vortex. Intense discussion of the long-suppressed event brought a sense of relief—a strong sense of catharsis—that would not have been possible without the clue of the energy blockage that I had picked up.

***Ron*** Ron is a clinical psychologist who specializes in working with AIDS patients. He finds Mind Clearing especially effective in diminishing the effects of neuropathy that often accompany this long-term disease. If the client cannot tolerate touch, because of pain or open sores, he unruffles the painful area in the field and does the Etheric Unruffle, including time for modulation of energy. In addition, he teaches the patients and their significant others to do some daily form of centering and connection of the chakras to maintain an open flow in the energy field. With each client he does a careful review of the stress levels and helps them to explore ways of diminishing pressure and tension in their daily lives. These changes in life patterns often require a release of faulty thinking and expectations, a process that is facilitated by working with the related chakra area. Control issues, for instance, relate to the solar plexus center that may feel empty or constricted without the defense of being in charge. As the client learns to keep the center open and activates the energy of the heart center, the need for control can diminish, be released, and soften into a more accepting personality style.

## Working through the Grief Process

The loss of a significant person is inevitable at some time or other in one's life. It has been said that all relationships end in either physical death or separation. It is, therefore, surprising that most people spend very little conscious effort preparing for death as a natural life event. The impact of a major loss can be lessened if the survivor is in otherwise good emotional health. However, if the loss comes at a time when there is already a deficit or significant blockage in the flow of *Qi*, it can have a devastating effect, disrupting the whole life pattern and emotional equilibrium.

Energetically, grief diminishes all of the chakras and the related fields. If there is underlying good health, the field may bounce back each day with a simple technique such as the Full Body Balance or the Chakra Meditation. The client

### JEAN'S STORY

Jean was a client who suffered immobility and depression because her mother was dying "by inches" in a nursing home over a period of many months. This kind of complicated loss, where the body is still alive but the mind is unclear and the personality altered, requires careful therapeutic support. The inevitable loss loomed like a monster before Jean, yet she had no way of preparing herself for it. Resolution of the tension required helping Jean to center on a daily basis and to express all the emotions associated with her mother, including anger about the mother's past alcoholism. Rebalancing of the energy field throughout this painful process was assisted by the Magnetic Unruffle and the comforting touch of the Full Body Connection.

Shortly before her mother's actual transition, Jean was able to connect with her own spiritual resources that allowed her to see the mother's slow dying as a path of learning and to connect with a wider, more transpersonal view of the dying process.

can learn to do this on a regular basis as a self-help technique (see chapter 17) to maintain energetic balance for the period of normal grieving that may last 1 to 2 years, depending on the significance of the loss. For people with more complex issues that have been triggered by the death, psychotherapy combined with balancing of the field is a good option.

## Dealing with Depression

As with grief, depression literally depresses and diminishes the entire energy field. The difference is that depression is more pathological, causing physical symptoms of sleeping and eating disturbances and emotional lability with inability to be enthusiastic about life. The field responds more slowly to energetic interventions especially if the depression is of more than a few weeks' duration as there is very little *Qi* available.

The Full Body Connection is usually helpful on a daily basis, and the Magnetic Unruffle is useful, if medication is indicated, to smooth the field and potentiate the effect of the antidepressant. Assessment of the chakras to find which one closes first after balancing the field may yield clues about the area that is most disturbed and in need of daily support, with affirmations and centering.

## TOM'S STORY

Tom, a businessman who was depressed for several months, experienced closing of the root chakra whenever he became angry. Because the anger could not be expressed safely in the competitive world of business, Tom's entire system would shut down and fill him with a vast sense of hopelessness and despair. Relief required awareness of the anger mechanism, finding safe outlets for his rage, and helping him to feel his body and enjoy life more fully. Initially, he did these things "just to get even" with his adversaries, but his actions put the blocked energy of the anger to work in a more constructive fashion that later gave him an increased sense of joy and vitality.

## Managing Bipolar Disorders

Bipolar disorders in which the patient cycles between elation and depression, or manic-depressive disorders, appear to have their source in chemical imbalance of the body. Response to medication, again, can be enhanced with systemic applications of Healing Touch that the client can learn as self-help techniques. The major impact of energetic work as a complement to treatment is the sense of self-control the client gains. Even the worst mood swing is not so overwhelming if the client knows how to unruffle his energy field, hold the chakras, and gently comfort the body.

## Overcoming Stress Reactions, Anxiety, and Phobias

Whereas depression affects approximately 20% of the population and bipolar disorders 1–2%, nearly everyone experiences stress reactions and anxiety (APA, 1998). This huge area of need can be treated with medication, but the power to overcome obstacles has to be activated within the client. As the person explores other ways of responding to difficult life situations, she may formulate new thinking patterns, sense the peacefulness of her spiritual base, and explore ways to release negative emotions quickly.

### KIMBERLY'S STORY

Kimberly worked in an office where the path to the rest room was directly in the line of sight of her supervisor. Every time she went to the rest room, she felt his piercing eyes evaluating her for wasting time. Her anxiety accelerated until she could not even imagine going to work without fear and trembling. Rather than lose her job, she decided to attend psychotherapy and resolve the conflict. In conjunction with desensitization, the therapist taught Kimberly imagery that would calm her, an affirmation or positive thought to repeat as needed, and to place her hands over the specific chakra areas of the body that felt most unprotected. Kimberly also learned how to smooth her energy field with the self-help techniques whenever she became anxious or fearful. She now is able to joke about imagining the boss's judgments of her rest room trips, helps her friends to stay centered in the office, and practices her own centering frequently.

## Hyperactivity in Children

An area of growing concern in the treatment field is the care of hyperactive children. Medication is often seen as the only or most expedient approach when, in fact, children respond very well to self-management techniques. Teaching a child to meditate or center is relatively easy provided that there is some skill in pacing to the child's interests. Examples from the popular culture like the *Karate Kid* or the imagery used by Olympic athletes can build a bridge for the child to value self-mastery. Beyond that, the Healing Touch approaches of unruffling,

Chakra Spread, and Mind Clearing give youngsters the opportunity to experience a calmer state of consciousness. Parents can easily reinforce the learning by offering these Healing Touch approaches on a daily basis. If nothing else, both the parents and child can gain a sense of power by dealing with their ongoing problems in a regular, caring, and systematic way. Of course, Healing Touch can easily be integrated into treatment plans that include medication and psychotherapy for hyperactivity.

## Assisting with Addictions Recovery

An addiction can be defined as an emotionally-backed demand for anything. This definition goes beyond the many forms of chemical dependency to include the hundreds of ways each of us may try to control others or obsess about what we think we want. These behavioral addictions are pervasive in every age group and cause untold social and personal distress. Highly addictive persons will often have major blockages in the second or third chakra areas. The depletion of energy in these major centers requires the individual to constantly seek ways of filling the void, even with substances or actions that are toxic or worsen the problem.

The key with an addictive personality is to help the individual find some way of taking personal control of the energetic imbalance. The 12-step programs give specific guidelines for self-help and day-by-day support through meetings within a spiritually oriented framework (Sparks, 1993). Similarly, the person needs day-by-day, sometimes hour-by-hour, rebalancing of the chakras and biofield, and reminders to connect with her Higher Power.

Touch, especially to smooth the field, is a quick and certain way of reconnecting with one's inner resources. In hospital settings, we have seen gentle, intentional touching calm the most frantic addictive cravings. A specific technique like Mind Clearing or the Chakra Spread can ease physical discomfort until the client can muster inner resources and move beyond the critical moment. The self-help techniques described in chapter 17 give further resources for self-empowerment.

# IMPLICATIONS FOR FAMILY THERAPY

Since Healing Touch creates a close emotional connection between practitioner and client, it is a natural device for helping families to bond. Work with couples can be enhanced by teaching them to share in sensing each other's energy fields, unruffling areas of pain, and exchanging a sequence like the Mind Clearing or the Full Body Connection. We recently worked with a couple in which the husband could not please his wife in any way. When he learned how to ease her migraine headaches using the Healing Touch approach—by unruffling the Pain Ridge—a whole new chapter opened in their relationship.

Working with energetic understanding allows families to welcome unborn babies as they sense the presence of the newcomer's energy field before birth.

Once the infant has arrived, the parents and older siblings have wonderful resources to calm baby fussiness with unruffling, modulation of energy to a specific site, and the Chakra Spread. As families grow older and their lives become more complex, the need for centering increases. Connection with the breath, setting the intent to hear each other, and working out problems with sensitivity to each person's energy field can do wonders for families in conflict.

Families constitute the largest interconnected energy field that most of us experience on a daily basis. Family therapists (Taub-Bynum, 1984) have begun exploring the family network of feelings, images, and energy as a powerful system called the Family Unconscious. With our specific understanding of the interactions between energy fields, the therapist can now work intentionally to balance the field of the entire family (Hover-Kramer & Shames, 1997, Ch 13).

# THE ADVENT OF COMPREHENSIVE ENERGY PSYCHOLOGY

Because the interface between energy approaches and psychotherapy is so compelling, it was only a matter of time until a fully developed new discipline of integrative, psychoenergetic practice would emerge. The publication of Dr. Fred Gallo's book *Energy Psychology* (1998) marked the introduction of this work to mainstream counselors and psychotherapists. In addition, Dr. Gallo has published new books ( Gallo, 2000; Gallo, 2002; Gallo & Vencenzi, 2000) that further elaborate his theoretical perspective of energy therapy, albeit mostly from the perspective of meridian-based treatment approaches. Furthermore, two research psychologists in the San Diego area produced a book that brought energy healing principles, addressing *Qi* flow patterns, to the general public (Lambrou & Pratt, 2000).

What was missing initially was the input from nurses and counselors who have practiced Healing Touch and Therapeutic Touch for many years using concepts of the biofield and chakras for emotional healing. To remedy this, two creative psychologist colleagues, Drs. David and Rebecca Grudermeyer, and the author joined forces to establish the Association of Comprehensive Energy Psychology in 1999. Since then, the organization has become very active in reaching healers involved with psychoenergetic balancing of the human vibrational matrix from many disciplines—addictions counselors, hypnotherapists, marriage/family counselors, mental health counselors, nurse clinicians, clinical social workers, chiropractors, acupuncturists, psychologists, and psychiatrists.

The reason that meridian-oriented therapies had become popular and more visible than biofield and chakra work in counseling is the presence of George Goodheart's work (described in Horowitz, 2001) with muscle testing in the early 1960s and Roger Callahan's (1985, 1996, 2001) work in dealing with emotional distress through tapping of the acupoints. Muscle tesing gave easy and scientific access to assessment of the client's inner psychoenergetic domain (Monti, D. et al., 1999) while Dr. Callahan popularized quick acupoint interventions in his books. The more comprehensive view of energy psychology is developing with a new well-organized, four level course (Grudermeyer, Grudermeyer, & Hover-Kramer, 2001) by the co-founders of the Association. It will be exciting to see the developments in this new discipline as conferences are held nationally and internationally and an active research base is developing and begins to be published.

## SUMMARY

Obviously, these are just indications for ways therapists might choose to work to enhance their practice. Energy-based concepts allow the counselor to comprehend the profound mystery that takes place in therapeutic exchanges. There seems to be a transfer of energy from the more centered intent of the helper to the less organized or depleted energy field of the client. We might say that the client's field begins to resonate to the higher harmony of the therapist's more intentional field. This transfer of energy is multidimensional — encompassing the emotional, mental, intuitive — and occurs mostly outside of conscious awareness. The more the psychotherapist brings field interactions into his awareness, the more he can monitor his own field and note subtle energetic changes in the client.

## REFERENCES

American Psychiatric Association (APA). (1998). *Diagnostic and statistical manual of mental disorders*, (DSM IV). Washington, DC: A.P.A. Press.

Association for Comprehensive Energy Psychology website—energypsych.org.

Callahan, R. (1985). *The five minute phobia cure*. Wilmington, DE: Enterprise Publishing.

Callahan, R. (1996). *Thought field therapy and trauma*. Indian Wells, CA: TFT Training Center.

Callahan, R. (2001). *Tapping the healer within*. Lincolnwood, IL: Contemporary Books.

Gallo, F. (1998). *Energy psychology*. Pittsburgh, PA: CRC Press.

Gallo, F. (2000). *Energy diagnostic and treatment methods*. New York: W. W. Norton & Co.

Gallo, F. (ed.) (2002). *Applications of energy psychology in psychotherapy*. New York: W. W. Norton & Co.

Gallo, F. & Vincenzi, H. (2000). *Energy tapping*. New York: W. W. Norton & Co.

Grudermeyer, D., Grudermeyer, R. & Hover-Kramer, D. (2001). *Individualized energy psychotherapy* ™ Level I & II notebooks. DelMar, CA: Willingness Works Press.

Holmes, T., & Rahe, R. (1967). The social readjusment rating scale. *Journal of Psychosomatic Research, XI*, 213–218.

Horowitz, J. M. (April 16, 2001). The man with magic fingers. *Time*, 65.

Hover-Kramer, D. and Shames, K. H. (1997). *Energetic approaches to emotional healing*. Albany, NY: Delmar.

Lambrou, P. & Pratt, G. (2000). *Instant emotional healing*. New York: Broadway Books.

Monti, D. A., Sinnott, J. & Kunkel, E. J. S. (1999). Muscle test responses to congruent and incongruent self-referential statements." *Perceptual and Motor Skills, 88*, 1019–1028.

Pert, C. (1997). *Molecules of emotion*. New York: Charles Scribner's Sons.

Rossi, E. L. (1986). *The psychobiology of mind body healing*. New York: W. W. Norton Co.

Sparks, T. (1993). *The wide open door*. Center City, MN: Hazelden Educational Materials.

Taub-Bynum, E. B. (1984). *The family unconscious*. Wheaton, IL: The Theosophical Publishing House.

# SECTION V

## Self-Care of the Practitioner

*A vital part of all caregiving is the clarity of the healer. In this part we will explore how Healing Touch interventions can be used for your self-care and how you can begin dialogue with the subconscious parts of yourself to increase self-knowledge. It is axiomatic that the more we know and understand ourselves the more we can be genuinely available to know and understand others. As part of the practitioner self-care emphasis we also offer a summary of courses available through the Healing Touch program.*

# CHAPTER 16

# New Developments in Healing Touch: Expansion of Resources for Practitioners

*Sharon Scandrett-Hibdon, Ph.D, RN*

> *"Healing and caring [are] seen within relationships, with caring presence as the potential vehicle for healing."*
>
> —C.L. Montgomery, 1993

## INTRODUCTION

As Healing Touch practitioners worked with their skills in energy healing over the past ten years, wider applications began to emerge. The deepening use of Healing Touch brought about a series of courses, in addition to the basic training, that allowed experienced teachers to further develop their ideas and create new integration with other knowledge bases. Some of the courses focus on applications of energy practice in specialized situations while others promote further refinement of practitioner skills. As holistic practitioners, the Healing Touch community believes in continuing, lifelong development of oneself and one's skills. This emphasis permeates the "Healing Touch Special Programs," some of which will be described here.

A number of opportunities are available to advanced students of Healing Touch. Several course offerings allow the practitioner to learn advanced energy interventions. Other courses enhance knowledge of energy anatomy. Still others develop communication skills, the use of hypnosis, and counseling skills. One practitioner took the Healing Touch concepts and translated them into Judeo-Christian language in order to reach persons within religious disciplines. Others have developed resources for releasing attachments, and combining Healing Touch with the practice of *Qigong*. And, moving into a whole new dimension of healing, a talented practitioner took the basic Healing Touch work and applied it to the healing of animals. This resulted in whole new audiences of Healing Touch fans, the "two-legged" and the "four-legged" ones. Let's explore some of these fascinating programs in more depth now.

# ADVANCED ENERGETIC INTERVENTIONS

The courses called "Advance Practice Series" offer refinement and expansion of the basic Healing Touch techniques described in section III. The two-course series was developed by Janet Mentgen, the identified founder of Healing Touch. She designed the program to continue energetic skill development of the healer. In the first course, basic Healing Touch interventions are refined to bring greater depth to the work. For example, autogenic relaxation is combined with the Full Body Connection to promote deeper relaxation while balancing the biofield. Techniques for the back are presented in further detail. The Sacred Chakra Spread enhances the simpler form of the Chakra Spread described in this book. Other energetic approaches are developed in response to specific questions and needs expressed within the classroom.

In the second course of Advance Practice, trauma release techniques for clearing memories of physical trauma are given. This is a very helpful intervention to clear the hurt of early trauma (Wardell, 2000). Case management issues based on an energetic approach are also explored. Practical protocols for issues participants bring to the course are designed in the classroom via case studies.

Another series of five advanced courses called "Energetic Healing" focuses on pracititioner healing. Developed by Dr. Mary Jo Bulbrook, this work provides a holistic approach to energy work. Beginning with an individual in-depth analysis of one's personal energy system, interventions are taught to facilitate physical, emotional, mental, and spiritual healing by clearing blockage in the biofield. The course then leads the practitioner to identify and release wounds which are stored in the human energy system. Participants examine ways of altering energetic disturbances to more functional patterns. The next class focuses on the outer layers of the biofield where beliefs appear to be held energetically. As personal healing evolves, relationships are explored, utilizing awareness of the chakras. Changing relationships energetically is the goal of succeeding classes, where participants change the vital life force that impacts relationships. Reshaping of family energy patterns weaves in work in changing family dynamics. Family patterns are explored to bring about healthier dynamics and expression. Dr. Bulbrook's notebooks (2000a; 2000b) give specific healing stories and demonstrate the effectiveness of this integrative approach.

# BUILDING COMMUNICATION SKILLS

Another series, the "Therapeutic Communication" course, blends energy work with effective counseling skills. Developed by this author, who saw the need for basic counseling skills in practitioners, the course provides the participants the tools to assist cognitive and emotional aspects that often surface when a client is receiving energy healing. Being aware of effective communication is as important as the ability to realign energy field disturbance. Healing is comprised of important cognitive functions—to *see*, *honor*, and *release* the energetic blocks that are no longer effective for the client.

The skills learned in Therapeutic Communication provide the practitioner with ways of exploring with the client his deeper patterns and core wounding. Reconnecting the emotions with cognitive beliefs provides information that permits clients to experience themselves and to have a perspective from which they can evaluate their lives. With such clarity, clients can make conscious choices to differentiate aspects of life that work from those that need to be altered. The basic counseling skills offered provide a supportive resource so that the energetic practitioner can gently assist the client in gaining personal insight.

The material of the course is based on the counseling theories of Truax and Carkhuff (1976) and Egan (1994). What differentiates this approach from traditional counseling, and makes it elegant, is that it gives clients full power to "call the shots," pacing their own work and changes as they are ready. This means that the practitioner must be detached from expecting outcomes and let the client's own healing process guide the interaction. Differing from many approaches in which the practitioner is considered the expert, this is a co-creative process, with the client leading the way. The practitioner acts as a guide to assist the client to expand awareness of a greater variety of options. Most of us use tunnel vision when we are distressed and think of only one or two possible choices. The greatest healing we can offer a client is to instill self-respect, something this approach offers, empowering the client to make his own decisions and to institute change at his own pace.

Another benefit of this training is consideration of the basic character structure and defense patterns as identified by well-known healer Barbara Brennan (1988; 1993). These defense patterns can be identified by their typical energetic structures and provide the client with information about his stress mechanisms and responses to trauma. They can be brought into balance through repatterning of the energy system which allows coping reactions to be more effective and creative.

This work is also very helpful to expand the self-awareness of the Healing Touch practitioner. One participant writes, "When I owned my own character structure, I was able to fit so many pieces together; it made sense to me why some things were hard, where I braced and protected myself, and why some things did not connect for me. Once this awareness came, I was able to directly override the basic defense posture. As I gained strength in positive experiences, I find the basic defense position carries less pull to act in old habitual ways. Dealing with this core material consciously has helped me also to be more compassionate with clients as they attempt to heal their own defense posture."

In addition, the course also takes the practitioner into constructive problem solving, an aspect designed to prevent treatment failures. Effective problem solving actively involves the practitioner, in contrast to other parts of the Therapeutic

Communication model. The practitioner must be planning and troubleshooting with clients to ensure that clients accomplish the desired goals.

An extension of the Therapeutic Communication work is a course called "Healing Touch in Relationships." The focus of this course is to bring energy concepts and effective communication tools into one's daily life through relatedness. Often our most precious relationships require that we have new ways of establishing closeness and enriching communication. Communication skills that deepen the connections between partners are taught. These skills are then supported by energetic techniques which deepen intimacy and bring both individuals into balance. Conflict resolution and "holding space" for one's partner are also practiced. An additional benefit of this course is that Healing Touch is taught to be delivered in a loving way so that greater understanding and support for each partner can occur.

Another course focuses on the use of hypnosis in conjunction with Healing Touch. Developed by psychologist, Dr. Clare Etheridge, and Janet Mentgen, the course is called "Words that Heal: Using Hypnosis with Healing Touch." It offers the practitioner natural ways of bridging with the subconscious through the use of trance states and story telling. This assists the client to remember old events that can then be released in a loving and supportive environment as they emerge. Study of the effectiveness of words upon healing states is explored (Watkins, 1987). Participants learn the use of relaxation, imagery, pain interventions, self-hypnosis, and reframing. Each level of the course offers deeper levels of understanding about hypnosis and the development of the healer. Many practitioners have found this course useful in developing their work, as it offers them a way to carefully deal with the client's painful material that may spontaneously emerge in a session.

## ENHANCING PRACTITIONER RESOURCES

Often, as a need for a practitioner resource becomes identified in the Healing Touch community, a teacher comes forth to meet the challenge. Sue Hoveland is such a person. She saw the need for increased understanding of human anatomy and physiology in nurses who had not studied the material recently. Also, she noticed that non-nurse participants often had limited anatomical knowledge. Thus, she developed a course entitled "Experiential Anatomy and Physiology for Healers." With a wide background in massage, neuromuscular therapy, craniosacral therapy, and Axiatonal Alignment, she was the natural person to develop this course. She teaches awareness of anatomy that HT practitioners can use to assist client to release tension from their bodies deeply and quickly. She has developed new physical energy treatments that build on the foundational Healing Touch treatments. Awareness about the body gained from this training facilitates the practitioner's own healing as well. For example, learning to sense the different organs of the body is part of the learning experience (Gosling, et al., 1997). As awareness increases, the healer's personal health improves. Another outcome of the lively training classes is that practitioners learn specifically how to work with affected organs and systems. Sue reports, "Energetically cleansing the liver can bring up old anger for release as it clears out toxins on all levels. It has helped some clients with hepatitis C to normalize their liver enzymes (Hoveland, 1999, p.8).

Other practitioners have taken Healing Touch into interesting settings with special populations. Damaris Jarboux went to China and studied with *Qigong* master teachers. Exchange of assessment and intervention techniques has resulted in both groups wishing to work together more fully (Jarboux, 1999, p. 11) and Jarboux teaches a combination of the Chinese energy technique with the more Western-oriented Healing Touch. Another practitioner, Kathy Sinnett, has developed a course focusing on "Spirit Release" (Sinnett, 1999, p. 9). This work allows for removal of harmful entities that may have entered during a time of psychic openness, such as trauma, while under the influence of drugs or anesthesia, or during extreme fear. The clearing possible with this work has profound effects on freeing the soul (Moody, 1993; Eliade, 1964).

One physical therapist uses Healing Touch in an aquatic environment in which she treats handicapped children and adults. She reports phenomenally deep relaxation and ease of movement as she clears and modulates energy with clients in the swimming pool. Another group of nurses uses Healing Touch in an inner city setting helping young women who affiliate in gangs to deal with their anger and rage. Staff in an Alzheimer's unit found that daily treatments with Healing Touch brought brief moments of lucidity and calming to the often agitated and confused patients. We could describe the applications of energy healing in hundreds of other settings: applications and opportunities to learn are as wide as our human creativity will allow.

# HEALING TOUCH FOR ANIMALS

"Healing Touch for Animals" is a workshop that teaches owners of pets and horses to assist their animal friends energetically. Founder of the program Carol Komitor writes as follows (personal communication, 2001):

> The recognition of a need for an animal related Healing Touch class came to me as I was teaching and answering question after question about animal energies. Throughout my early Healing Touch career, the central office was referring animal questions to me, tapping into my 13-year background as a veterinary technician. All the questions made me realize there was a need for energetic care for our animal population.
>
> When I made a commitment to search out this new workshop possibility, animal teachers literally came to me. They quickly started coming one

after another as if presenting themselves through a revolving door. Techniques began developing as I addressed their needs and soon, enough information was ready to share with interested two-leggeds wanting to work with their four-legged friends.

The folks in the cutting horse community, with whom I had worked extensively, urged me to travel to Texas and teach them how to work with their horses. They had seen the results of my work in their horses during healing from injuries and illness, as well as during competitions. The first Healing Touch for Animals workshop was launched in 1996. This was the beginning of an unbelievable mushrooming of interest in this work. The interest came from Healing Touch practitioners and students, but the work was also reaching a different population of animal lovers who were unfamiliar with energy concepts.

There are three animal teachers who have given me the majority of information and I honor them in the logo of the program. Delite was a cutting horse that first came to me because of a major leg injury that virtually ended her competitions. After extensive healing treatments and veterinary care, Delite returned to winning status in her competitions.

Golden retriever Bogart Smith, CTD (certified training dog), was a retired sight-assistant canine who traveled with me early in the program as a demonstration dog. Bogart, like all service dogs, took his job seriously. He would wear his service cape as we boarded an airplane, find a comfortable place at my feet during the ride, and make the trips look easy. As Bogart went to work in classes, he would energetically connect with each of the canine participants in the workshop. He gave me understanding of ways animals communicate with each other intuitively, without words.

The third animal teacher was my cat Pokey Joe, a member of my family unit for 18 years. He allowed me to see how animals connect with people and gave me awareness of the multitudes of animal healers. Pokey would go to the chakra in need to help his two-legged counterpart. He would place his paws on the chakra, and then utilize his purring mechanism to help the chakra to open. He knew who needed assistance in the classroom and helped me to recognize the animal healers in each workshop.

My vision for the future is to integrate this program more into the veterinary medicine curricula, to train trainers how to embrace the energy of competitions and to give those who love a pet a new understanding of their animal friend. I continue to hear wonderful stories of how lives, both of the animals and the humans, have been changed as students embrace this work. The program promotes the oneness of all creatures and our relationship to the environment. This work can cause healing at all possible levels. I am blessed to be able to do the work I love and to assist others in embracing this aspect of healership.

(Further information about this fascinating program can be obtained through the listing given in Appendix B.)

Several other HT practitioners have reported working in wild animal shelters in their communities to connect with and support the healing of animals from the wilderness. Besides helping to facilitate rest and the acceptance of nutrition, the energy work seems to calm animals and speed trust-building so they can receive adequate medical care. More research and documentation of HT with animals is needed and will undoubtedly emerge as the field expands.

# HEALING TOUCH SPIRITUAL MINISTRY PROGRAM

The Spiritual Ministry program is now an affiliate of the Colorado Center for Healing Touch, standing on its own as an interpretation of energy healing concepts in Judeo-Christian language. Linda Smith, founder, writes, "The program was born three and a half years ago to answer the unique needs of those who wish to learn hands-on healing for church and spiritual ministry settings. The program appeals especially to parish nurses and nurses. . . wishing to understand the laying on of hands and other Healing Touch techniques. The program also appeals to ministers from all denominations as well as chaplains and the lay community who seek to explore a spiritual healing ministry. The aim of the program is to help bring back healing into our faith communities and ministry/service settings everywhere" (Smith, 1999, p. 9).

The content of the courses in the program parallel those of the regular Healing Touch program but are framed in Judeo-Christian language. The history of healing in Jewish and Christian traditions is presented, giving the foundation for Healing Touch as an act of service to others within one's faith. Each course is taught with a spiritual focus. Biblical explanations and quotes are used to assist students in understanding the nature of healing (Smith, 2000). Personal spiritual development is emphasized so that the healer can continue to receive more energy and guidance from the unlimited Source of all energy. The program is reaching leaders within churches, and Linda has recently presented at the Pontifical Institute of Priests of Pastoral Theology for Health Care in Rome.

# SUMMARY

From the brief overview presented herein, the reader may catch the excitement of those working in Healing Touch and allied energy healing work. In seeing the many applications of energy concepts, we recognize that much more will develop as practitioners develop their unique skills and creativity. This is only the beginning of the potential and richness of this work. As we expand our human awareness, many more of possibilities will unfold. Look at what has been developed in the ten short years that Healing Touch began as a localized training that expanded nationally and internationally. We can only imagine the depth of further work that will evolve because the potential is as wide as our creative talents will take us.

# REFERENCES

Brennan, B. A. (1988). *Hands of light.* New York: Bantam Books.

Brennan, B. A. (1993). *Light emerging.* New York: Bantam Books.

Bulbrook, M. J. (2000a). *Healing stories, giving and receiving, teaching and learning energy-based therapy.* Lakewood, CO: Healing Touch Partnerships.

Bulbrook, M. J. (2000b). *Healing touch notebook.* Lakewood, CO: Healing Touch Partnerships.

Egan, G. (1994). *The skilled helper.* Pacific Grove, CA: Brooks/Cole.

Eliade, M. (1964). *Shamanism: Archaic techniques of ecstasy.* Princeton, NJ: Princeton University Press.

Gosling, J. A., Harris, P. F., Humpherson J. R., Whitmore I., & Wiullan, P. T. (1997). *Human anatomy coloring book.* New York: Mosby-Wolfe.

Hoveland, S. (Nov., 1999). The birth of an anatomy class. *Healing Touch Newsletter . 9* (4), 8.

Hover-Kramer, D., Mentgen, J. and Scandrett-Hibdon, S. (1986). *Healing touch.* Albany, NY: Delmar.

Jarboux, D. (Nov., 1999). Quigong and healing touch in China. *Healing Touch Newsletter. 9* (4), 11.

Montgomery, C. L. (1993). *Healing through communication: The practice of caring.* Newberry Park, CA: Sage Publications, 36.

Moody, R. (1993). *Reunions.* New York: Villard Books.

Schoen, A. M., and Proctor, P. (1995). *Love, miracles and animal healing.* New York: Simon & Schuster.

Schwartz, C. (1996). *Four paws and five directions.* Berkeley, CA: Celestial Arts.

Sinnett, K. (Nov., 1999). How I got where I am now. *Healing Touch Newsletter, 9* (4), 8-9.

Smith, L. (Nov., 1999). Healing touch spiritual ministry flies on its own! *Healing Touch Newsletter, 9* (4), 9-10.

Smith, L. L. (2000). *Called into healing: Reclaiming our Judeo-Christian legacy of healing touch.* Arvada, CO: Healing Touch Spiritual Ministry (HTSM) Press.

Truax, C. B., and Carkhuff, R. R. (1967). *Toward effective counseling and psychotherapy: Training and practice.* Chicago, IL: Aldine Press.

Wardell, D. (Feb., 2000). Trauma release. *Complementary and Alternative Therapies. 6* (1), 17–20.

Watkins, J. G. (1987). *Hypnotherapeutic techniques.* New York: Irvington Publishers.

# CHAPTER 17

# Healing Touch for the Caregiver

*"Good thoughts don't make a heaven, any more than they make a garden. . . . We are to learn first what is heaven, and secondly, how to make it. We are to ascertain what is right and then how to perform it."*

—Florence Nightingale in Calabria & Macrae, 1994

## INTRODUCTION

There is a wide discrepancy between the talk about self-care and actual research or hands-on practice in support of this concept. For instance, all nursing curricula teach the nurse to be a caregiver, but few single courses in our current curricula address the needs of the caregiver. Attention to self-care is even less evident when caregivers begin their professional careers and need supportive mentoring.

## THE NEED FOR SELF-CARE

With their many good intentions for helping others, caregivers are often least likely to pay attention to their own needs. This may be due to an outgoing, altruistic focus or to an internal dynamic of avoiding or discounting personal needs. Whatever the mechanism, caregivers are at high risk for stress, tension-related illness, and what is being called "burn-out."

Several publications address the issues of healing arts practitioners. Caryn Summers (1992) writes about the high-risk environments in which the largest group of professional caregivers—nurses—work. She estimates that more than 80% of nurses suffer from codependency—that is, they are overly concerned with pleasing others, often to their own detriment. Chemical addiction rates are 30 times greater for nurses than for the general population (Summers, 1992, p. 105). Similar conclusions were described by two nurses who summed up the caregiver dilemma in the title of their book, *I'm Dying to Take Care of You* (Snow & Willard, 1989). Large institutions like hospitals seem to generate and support dysfunctional, addictive patterns, causing many idealistic caregivers to become bogged down in the mire of bureaucracy and impossible expectations (Schaef &

Fassel, 1988). The experience of being a wounded healer and the long road to recovery is described in Jarrett's (1993) book, *Caring for the Caregiver*. Her extensive bibliography leads the reader to a variety of self-help strategies.

Self-care is becoming a highly valued commodity in a time when high technology and the sheer volume of human need inundate the health care scene. Somehow, to recapture the essence of our vision as caregivers in any of the helping professions, we must return to our own humanity as the locus of healing. Unfortunately, there are few guidelines, or academic curricula, for achieving this valuable quality which is the basis for offering our healing presence to others.

While research demonstrates the importance of self-transcendence for our clients to achieve optimum functioning (Reed, 1996, 1992), few caregivers apply such ideas to themselves. Beyond learning what is good for our clients, we as healing practitioners must apply the information we have learned to ourselves. A shift in perception is required: the principles of Healing Touch—attention to body, mind, spirit, early intervention, frequent centering, and inward focusing—are resources for us as individuals to use. This is the journey to a holistic perspective, central to the philosophy of Slater et al. (1999) and the rich volume *Holistic Nursing* (Dossey, et al., 2000). Becoming a Healing Touch practitioner, thus, is not just about learning the techniques and concepts described in sections II and III but about the use of self and the practice of presence, not only what we *do* but who we *are*.

Becoming a Healing Touch practitioner is a transformative experience. Dr. Norma Geddes, among the first to study this process in depth, states "It is a process of making changes in all facets of life based on a perception of the self as a unitary, spiritual, self-caring, and self-nurturing individual" (personal communication, May, 2001).

In this chapter we will explore applications of Healing Touch concepts to the caregiver and in the next, guidelines for personal development of the practitioner.

## ESSENTIALS OF ENERGY-ORIENTED SELF-CARE

The essentials of energetic self-care require ongoing attentiveness to the quality and state of the personal biofield. One method used by persons recovering from addictions is a personal check-in technique called HALT. This is a reminder to ask oneself, right now am I Hungry? am I Angry? am I Lonely? am I Tired? In this way, a simple acronym becomes a means for internal self-assessment that can be prescriptive for relief interventions. In a similar vein, we can use PEMS to assess the Physical, the Emotional, the Mental, and the Spiritual dimensions of the biofield.

The physical body requires nutrition, activity, and rest. If we work with it proactively and caringly, it lasts longer and self-heals more capably than any man-made device. Self-knowledge is the key to effective physical care since every organism is a unique combination of heredity, life events, and personal mechanisms. We must learn not only to rest, but how often, how long, and how to assess when we are tired. We must learn the kind of exercise that is optimal for our body-type. We must learn how much to eat, when to eat, and when to stop.

The emotional body can predominate all other aspects of awareness when it is in disarray. Strong negative emotions require prompt attention and assistance, just as would be required for a physical symptom. Moving toward positive supportive emotions is an integral part of our human journey toward personal fulfillment.

Mental states, as exemplified by our thought patterns, can also overwhelm us if they are destructive, judgmental, or critical. Such patterns can even harm the physical body or cause emotional depression, as demonstrated in the vast literature showing mind/body interactions. The practice of helpful thought patterns and peaceful images can do much to assist the body and emotions, as we shall see in the next chapter.

Self-assessment of the spiritual dimension may require something as simple as being still, and listening to the inner voice. The practices of centering required in all healing work readily move us to this new perspective—nothing is quite as demanding, or as immediate, as it seems in the moment.

While there are many books available on working with one's inner life, few delineate how to best to utilize self-help classes and methods. The reader is encouraged to explore resources such as psychologists David and Rebecca Grudermeyer's *Sensible Self-Help* (1996) for a definitive road map on the personal healing journey.

## HEALING TOUCH FOR SELF-CARE

The question is, then, who cares for the caregiver? Obviously, it must be ourselves as we look at the tremendous challenges and risks we handle on a daily basis. In our Healing Touch classes we have found that the techniques offer significant tools and starting points for self-awareness and self-nurturing. The hands-on approach of Healing Touch offers practical, powerful methods that go beyond mental control or imagery. Self-healing is essential for transferring the focused, intentional energy that is needed to do Healing Touch with others. In the succeeding exercises we will explore self-healing work. Follow along and develop your own approaches to begin a program of genuine care of the caregiver—you.

### Heart Centering

Each caregiving intervention begins with centering. This requires you to move within yourself to find an inner reference point or core. In contacting this inner core, you begin to find stillness and peacefulness and a sense of being unified, integrated, and focused. Centering also implies being totally present in the immediate moment and developing the ability to refocus any time the mind becomes distracted. Naturally, this requires regular practice, preferably two to three times a day for at least 15 to 20 minutes, to quiet the busy mind, relax the body, and calm the emotions. When you as a caregiver have achieved the practice of centering, you will be able to work easily in most difficult situations. As a bonus, others around you may sense your calmness and move to their own centered states of awareness more readily.

One of the most critical elements of centering is, of course, knowing when you are *not* in a peaceful state of mind. At first, practitioners seem to find this difficult to do because they attend mentally to the needs of the client rather than to their own internal state. Invariably, when a student of Healing Touch tells her mentors that a technique did not work, we find that centering has not been done completely enough. So we encourage potential healers to practice centering every time they feel the slightest emotional distress during the workday. The emotions are like sensors, like antennae, that allow us to receive quick feedback when something is amiss.

It is important to center from the heart chakra, the energy vortex that allows us to feel compassion and unconditional love. In using the heart-centered energy for self-healing we can also allow compassion to flow toward ourselves. Heart centering can be done several times a day until it becomes an automatic response in each difficult situation. Once you become attuned to self-caring, you will readily detect when you are not centered because the inner voices will be judgmental and harsh. Remember, our minds and bodies have a tremendous capacity to respond to the positive suggestions we can make, especially from a centered state of consciousness.

Studies of biofeedback (Othmer, et al., 1999) show that ordinary consciousness is characterized by the beta brain wave pattern; centering shifts brain wave activity to alpha, a slower, more focused pattern. The alpha brain wave frequency allows us to increase perception and to develop our intuitive skills more readily.

## EXERCISE

## HEART CENTERING

1. Begin by allowing your awareness to move to your heart center. . . . Take a slow, deep breath and feel the energy of compassion and caring. . . . As you exhale, visualize the tension and stress in your body flowing out your hands and feet. . . . Do this three times. . . . Releasing. . . . Letting go.

2. Visualize an emerald green light at the heart center. . . . Feel the sensation of warmth and balance move into your chest . . . shoul-

*(continues)*

*(continued)*

ders . . . arms . . . head . . . abdomen . . . thighs, legs, and feet. . . . Relax the entire body. . . . If the mind wanders, refocus at the heart center and repeat the process.

3. See with your inner eye a friend or someone you wish to help. Sense your heart center opening to the person in front of you and note how good it feels to send out the vibration of caring.

4. Allow the person in front of you to be yourself, perhaps as a little child or at a time that was difficult, a time you were embarrassed or upset about something.

5. Allow that same quality of love and compassion you had for your friend to go to yourself. Forgive and feel the vibration of compassion. Allow yourself to learn from the difficult experience. Be very gentle with yourself.

6. Connect again with the breath and gently come back to full awareness.

## Chakra Meditation

Many practices access a meditative state, but actually moving the hands over the chakras to activate their energies increases the effect. This meditation may be appropriate early in the morning just on awakening when the body is still at rest and the mind is starting to arouse. It is also useful to do this practice whenever you are fatigued or discouraged as it allows you to feel the vital life force flowing through the body.

EXERCISE

### CHAKRA MEDITATION

1. Set your intention for the healing you wish for yourself. Begin to mobilize the healing forces within by identifying what you want to heal or release.

2. Begin with the spine in alignment, either lying down or sitting up in a comfortable position. Celebrate your aliveness with a positive statement such as, "I feel my joy; vitality is now flowing through me; I deserve love and now attract loving thoughts."

3. Releasing any tension with the out-breath, allow the hands to move over the root chakra area. . . . Feel your life force, your sense of belonging on the earth, your sense of safety and security with your-

*(continues)*

*(continued)*

    self. Hold each position for 1 to 3 minutes depending on your sense of what is needed in each area.

4. Move both hands over the sacral chakra. . . . Sense your body in balance; sense your emotional nature, and make note of any current feeling for later attention, and release what is not needed at this time.

5. Move the hands over the solar plexus area. . . . Notice how good it feels to protect this vulnerable area. Allow yourself to take in energy from the universe in the form of golden sunlight, wind, or ocean waves. . . . Sense your ability to be assertive and effective in communicating with others.

6. Move both hands to the heart center. . . . Feel the flow of unconditional love toward others; feel their love flowing into you. Send out the flow of this love to yourself, forgiving easily and learning from all past experiences. Feel the support of the three lower centers as you do this.

7. Move the hands to the throat center. . . . Sense your ability to express your being; enjoy singing, chanting, making sounds, speaking with clarity.

8. Proceed to the brow center, the intuitive chakra. . . . Sense your awareness expanding, able to see with insight and wisdom. See all there is to see; sense what another person's situation might be. Allow yourself an insight about a current situation.

9. Reach to the crown chakra, feeling your connection with the Infinite. . . . Unlimited resources of love and wisdom are available to you through this connection.

10. Slowly relax the hands, continuing to feel your energy flow as you move forward and set your intent for the next activity of the day.

## Connecting the Chakras

There are many ways of enhancing one's sense of well-being by connecting the energy centers of the major joints with the chakras related to the spinal column. One way is to follow the basic outline called "Chakra Connections" given by Brugh Joy (1979, pp. 269–274) and to personalize this exercise by adding your own variations.

The following exercise is a variation that we have found helpful. This needs to be done with a centered state of consciousness in a time frame that allows all parts of your energy system to integrate the experience. Many of our students do this practice before arising in the morning or on a break in the work schedule when they need an energy boost.

EXERCISE

## CHAKRA SELF-CONNECTION

1. Begin by acknowledging your connection with the supportive Universe and sensing your inner center. Set your intention for the help you need.

2. Feeling the energy of the breath in your lungs and heart center, gently let it go to the arms and hands, then connect both hands above and below the foot on the nondominant side.

3. Move the hands higher, connecting the ankle to the knee. Hold until you feel a flow of warmth or a pulsation, a sense of aliveness, moving from the ankle to the knee.

4. Move the hands to connect the knee and hip, holding until you feel the warming flow.

5. Connect in similar fashion on the dominant side the foot, ankle and knee, knee and hip.

6. Connect both hips by letting energy flow through the hands to the hips.

7. Connect the root chakra, with one hand below or on the perineum and the other on the sacral center, just below the umbilicus.

8. When there is a flow of vitality from the feet through the lower abdomen, move higher by placing one hand on the sacral center and the other on the solar plexus. You will know exactly how much holding you need in this vulnerable area to recharge your batteries and to feel genuinely nurtured.

9. Feeling the support of all the lower centers, connect the solar plexus and heart center sensing the flow of unconditional love toward others and yourself.

10. With one hand on the heart let the other hand connect to the wrist, the elbow, the shoulder. Alternate so that the other hand is on the heart center and you connect the other wrist, elbow, and shoulder.

11. Place both hands on both shoulders giving yourself a nice big hug. Remember that all we do for ourselves is an extension of the gifts of Universal Love, of which there is a limitless supply.

*(continues)*

*(continued)*

12. Connect the heart chakra and the throat center, the throat and the brow, the brow and the crown. Finally, connect the crown and the transpersonal point above the crown to celebrate your connection with Higher Power as you understand it. Feel the boundaries of your marvelous energy being that extends out about as far as your hands can reach. And now, you are ready for whatever is next on your agenda!

## Brush Down and Shake Out

Often, we find ourselves in situations where tension is palpable and the energy feels heavy, as when a caregiver enters a hospital room full of angry family members. Remaining centered before, during, and after such an encounter requires consummate skill. Simply brushing down your own biofield to calm the jangled emotions and smooth the jagged edges of the field can be very helpful. This brushing may be a few sweeps through the entire field, head to toe, while taking some deep breaths or a smoothing of the field over such chakras that seem most vulnerable, as the heart, solar plexus, or sacral centers.

A similar ritual is to release stagnated or sticky energy by shaking out hands and feet and moving the body in a healthy wiggle. Needless to say, these techniques may best be done away from persons who might not understand or misinterpret what we're doing.

Another option, of course, is to do a similar process mentally, visualizing your hands moving in the areas as needed. The intent is always one of providing genuine caring for self in the hundreds of difficult times that you face as a health caregiver and doing it quickly, as close in time to the triggering event as possible.

## Personal First Aid

All the knowledge you have gained by learning techniques to help another person have practical applications for self-care. For instance, it is as natural to soothe a child's wound by unruffling the area over an injury as to soothe one's own wounds, burns, or cuts. The more specific technique of Ultrasound would speed healing in a concentrated area by helping an injury to mend. In more extensive injuries, such as bone fracture, repeated smoothing and modulation of *Qi* over the break can speed healing. Many practitioners report good success in applying Healing Touch techniques on themselves because they can repeat the treatments as often as necessary.

# LIMITATIONS OF SELF-HEALING

In our discussion of self-caring methods it is important to be clear about its limitations. The self-healing concepts work best as preventative or health maintenance tools, and they seem to be effective when utilized at the first symptom of discomfort or distress. It is self-evident that centering, a basic requirement for healing work, is difficult when symptoms are acute, such as with a migraine headache. Further, it is untenable to postpone medical treatment for any ongoing symptom that is not relieved quickly by energetic interventions.

Let yourself see Healing Touch as an adjunct, a complement to other treatment modalities, never as a cure-all or panacea for your emotional or physical ills. Physical symptoms that need medical care may be further helped by utilizing Healing Touch. For example, pain medication is potentiated by smoothing and balancing of the biofield.

Emotional symptoms, similarly, may release quickly with centering and some of the self-help concepts suggested previously. For example, early signs of irritability, restlessness, fatigue, or sadness may find relief with the centering and reconnecting to Higher Resources of the transpersonal perspective. However, energy-based concepts are no substitute for treatment of ongoing or severe symptoms such as panic disorder or depression. Good psychotherapy with skill on the part of the therapist and trust on the part of the client are needed to work out complex issues. Interestingly, we have found that such self-caring techniques as the Chakra Meditation can be very useful in alleviating the prevalent morning "blahs" in someone who is being treated for depression.

# SUMMARY

All healing work is ultimately self-healing work. Almost all Healing Touch techniques described in previous chapters can be used on oneself with the only difference being that the energetic contrast will be more subtle when working on oneself than when working with another person. Hopefully, all practitioners and clients will avail themselves of this tremendous resource for health maintenance and prevention.

Because of our interest in teaching self-care to others, we have a commitment as practitioners to learn from our own experience and to teach others from this personal understanding. Most importantly, as we apply our skills of self-caring, we are showing new possibilities to our many colleagues in need.

# REFERENCES

Calabria, M., & Macrae, J. (Eds.). (1994). *Suggestions for thought by Florence Nightingale.* Philadelphia: University of Pennsylvania Press, 8.

Dossey, B., Keegan, L., Guzzetta, C. (2000). *Holistic nursing: A handbook for practice*, 3rd ed., Gaithersburg, MD: Aspen Publication.

Geddes, N. (1999). *The nature of the experience of personal transformation in Healing Touch practitioners: A heuristic inquiry.* Unpublished doctoral dissertation, Virginia Commonwealth University, Richmond, VA.

Grudermeyer, D. & Grudermeyer, R. (1996). *Sensible self-help: The first road map for the healing journey.* DelMar, CA: Willingess Works Press.

Jarrett, R. M. (1993). *Caring for the caregiver.* Beaverton, OR: Happy Talk Books.

Joy, B. (1979). *Joy's way.* Los Angeles: J. P. Tarcher, Inc.

Othmer, S., Othmer, S. F., and Kaiser, D. A. (1999). EEG biofeedback. In Evans, J. R. and Abarbanel, A. (Eds.). *Introduction to quantitative EEG and neurofeedback.* San Diego, CA: Academic Press, 244–310.

Reed, P. G. (1992). An emerging paradigm for the investigation of spirituality in nursing. *Research in Nursing and Health, 15*, 349–357.

Reed, P. G. (1996). Transcendence: Formulating nursing perspectives. *Nursing Science Quarterly, 9*, 2–4.

Schaef, A. W., & Fassel, D. (1988). *The addictive organization.* San Francisco: Harper and Row.

Slater, V. E., Maloney, J. P., Krau, S. D., Eckert, C. A. (1999). Journey to holism. *Journal of Holistic Nursing, 17* (4), 346–364.

Snow, C., & Willard, D. (1989). *I'm dying to take care of you.* Redmond, WA: Professional Counselor Books.

Summers, C. (1992). *Caregiver, caretaker.* Mt. Shasta, CA: Commune-a-Key Publications.

# CHAPTER 18

# Self-Development of the Healing Touch Practitioner

> *"Applied to clinical situations, intuition is a component of complex judgment, the act of deciding what to do in a perplexing, often ambiguous and uncertain situation. It is the act of synthesizing empirical, ethical, aesthetic, and personal knowledge."*
>
> —Lynn Rew, 2000

## INTRODUCTION

Our discussion of the HT practitioner makes it clear that the energy field of the healer is the primary resource for healing. If we are free of emotional debris, we can be a connector or facilitator for the client in helping to make available the vast potential of the Universal Energy Field. If we are blocked in some way or out of balance, we cannot assist with this connection. In other words, there are no secrets in energy-based work: in the same ways that we sense the client's field with our Higher Sense Perception, so the client senses our ability to be fully present in the healing moment, or that we are distracted and unfocused.

In this chapter we will explore some of the major consideration for self-development that can provide ways to move more deeply into your inner awareness and develop your internal resources.

## THE INNER JOURNEY TO BECOMING A HEALING TOUCH PRACTITIONER

Over the past ten years, HT instructors have watched the fascinating journey of the starry–eyed beginner who is excited about helping others to the seasoned practitioner who is internally focused and deeply respectful of each client's personal healing process. For the certified HT practitioner, this transformation has some identifiable external markers, such as attending the three major weekend intensives (Level I, II-A, & II-B), the practitioner retreat that includes the beginning of a mentoring relationship (Level III-A), the practical work of selecting, assessing, and implementing interventions with 100 clients, careful documentation of all learning activities, and participation in the final practitioner retreat (Level III-B).

However, the inner journey to healership is as unique as each practitioner's vibrational energy pattern. It requires commitment to personal growth, self-understanding, integration of multi-level learning, and maturing. Little has been written about this aspect of healing practice. In the literature to date, Keegan and Dossey's (1998) warm book *Profiles of Nurse Healers* alludes to the complex inner journey of healing arts practitioners. Often, there are early childhood experiences that are coupled with a significant life event later on. These propel the individual to seek deeper levels of practice and greater personal understanding. In addition, B. Dossey et al. (1998) conducted a study of nurses to identify the knowledge and professional activities that lead to a nurse's becoming a holistically oriented practitioner. Most recently, Slater et al. (1999) undertook a study that identified the stages through which nurses move from their ordinary professional activities to a true embracing of holistic concepts, of which a most prominent feature is the dedication to self-care and personal development. While this study is not limited to HT practitioners, many of the case examples cited are nurse healers practicing HT. The context of holistic, integrative thinking appears to most effectively build the foundation for mature healership.

The authors of the study identify three major stages of development—*separation* from usual practice, a period of *marginality/liminality* in which new possiblities are explored, and *reintegration* (Slater et al., 1999). For some beginning HT practitioners, the separation stage may be simply attending weekend workshops, or basking in the retreat atmosphere of advanced classes. For others, there may be a total break with usual professional life; examples are the nurse who has left clinical practice altogether to find a new career, or the computer programmer who wishes to contribute to society at a more humanistic level. Once a sense of separation from more usual thinking has been achieved, new possibilities are explored. Seeing a *limen* as a threshold between two spaces allows us to consider this stage between separation and new integration as a time of liminality, or of liminal activity. This is often an awkward time in which the person may try out many new behaviors that appear unusual or confusing to friends and family. Nonetheless, this "in-between" period has definable steps that may or may not occur in sequential fashion. Through a grounded theory approach of qualitative research, Slater et al. (1999) were able to elicit in-depth responses from 18 selected holistic practitioners. The five recursive phases of self-change in the liminal stage were: a) information gathering, b) application (of new information) to others, c) refocus and self-change, d) application to self, and e) self-knowledge.

Before integration to new levels of understanding can occur, healing practitioners must journey through their own inner process. Becoming an HT facilitator involves much more of our personal selves than merely learning techniques and sharing them with others. The most significant shift in all seasoned practitioners is the refocus on true self-care and personal healing as the basis for reaching out to others. This chapter is an exploration of some of the many ways that we as practitioners can deepen our self-development. There are many additional resources beyond the scope of this text, and the reader is invited to peruse the rich resources for personal development cited in Dossey, Keegan & Guzzetta's third edition of *Holistic Nursing* (2000).

# PERSONAL DEVELOPMENT TECHNIQUES

The essential qualities of the healer, then, are a dedication to personal development, a commitment to keep gaining from experiences, an openness to new ideas, enthusiasm to take on the great adventure of life, and a willingness to work through personal difficulties with an attitude of flexibility.

Jung (1974), the great psychologist, said that the first part of our life is spent finding our personal identity, and the second part of life is moving into our greater identity as spiritual beings. He called this maturing *individuation* to differentiate from the achievement-oriented nature of our early life's work. Anyone who is serious about helping others needs to individuate—to be less dependent on outside opinions and be able to hear the inner guidance that is available through daily, committed practice.

## Journal Writing

One of the most effective ways to start the inner dialogue with the many layers of your inner being is by journal writing (journaling). A number of fine resource books are available to describe specific approaches (Cappachione, 1991; Progoff, 1975; Rainer, 1978), but the most important thing is to get started. It is helpful to have an attractive notebook that is available to you any time you wish to write and that is completely private. You might want to think of journal writing as writing letters to yourself as you begin to open dialogue with unknown aspects of yourself. As no new friendship could develop without regular communication, so this dialogue with the inner being, your own best friend, needs to be comfortable, enjoyable, and frequent.

The journal becomes a place for expressing feelings you may never have shared, for exploring ideas, or for reflecting on events in your life. This is not a clinical record or a log of daily activities, but rather a place to describe subjective experiences, images, gut reactions, future goals, and to celebrate an internal victory. Some people find it useful to use the journal to set the goals, intent, and energy for the day in the morning and then to review these items at the end of the day, noting what has been resolved and requires further action. Another way to increase your communication repertoire might be to write letters, which you don't necessarily send, to friends and adversaries. The key is creative self-expression while sensing the center of your being. The journal thus becomes a place where you experience your inner "home base."

## Dream Work

If journal writing provides an avenue for reaching out to the deeper self, dream work gives us windows into the inner world. To quote the great teacher, "Dream psychology opens a way to a general comparative psychology from which we may hope to gain the same understanding of the development and structure of the human psyche as comparative anatomy has given us concerning the human body" (Jung, 1974, p. 34). Although many dreams appear mysterious because of their symbolic nature, they are a self-portrait of something that is actually at work in the subconscious mind. Even a brief fragment or an emotion that we remember can give us some idea of the inner psyche and the unfolding self.

Some easy ways to track dreams and learn from the inner teacher are to set your intent to learn from a dream memory and have a pad, pen, and flashlight on hand when going to sleep. On awakening, write down the image, symbol, or emotional fragment before doing anything else, as activity disrupts the memory patterns. Even if you get only a small fragment, thank your inner being for the information. Remember that you are building a relationship with the unknown, deeper parts of yourself.

As you progress in getting more dream material, you may wish to sort out themes and patterns. This has to be done with the utmost respect since we know that any new friend would be frightened by criticism or judgment. Many books (Johnson, 1986; Thurston, 1978) give excellent tools for self-understanding through dream work.

### EXERCISE

### DREAM WORK

1. Begin by writing down as many key words associated with the dream as possible. Look at the key words you have written down and quickly make as many associations with each word as possible. For example, "woman" may be associated with mother, feminine, soft, comfort, old, wise, etc.

2. As you review the overall quality of the dream, certain associations will fit more precisely than others. There will be a sense of recognition. Note the associations that fit for the dream.

3. Begin to notice how the key words fit into a pattern, an overall observation or general statement that can be made, such as "The dreamer is always in some kind of trouble."

*(continues)*

*(continued)*

4. Allow yourself to think of ways this might be true for you and what message you can specifically draw from the statement.

5. Allow some action to follow. This may include writing down your insights, celebrating your awareness in some way, or doing something specific and practical as lighting a candle or putting a flower in a special place.

A colleague reported that she utilized this way of working with dreams. "In the early explorations of my own inner world," she states, "I had several repeated dreams about my car being out of control and some kind of fire in the rear end of it. I tried to look for associations with control issues but found no resolution that fit. After the dream kept repeating, I moved to action and took the car to a garage for a long overdue checkup and found that the brake linings, especially in the rear, were almost totally burned out."

It is interesting to note that many of our students report dreams of doing or learning HT. The healing archetype, as it is exemplified in HT, is very much alive in our troubled world. One dreamer described in detail learning how to do the Chakra Spread technique before it was presented in the classroom. Another student spoke of many regrets about not being at her mother's bedside at the time of the mother's transition. In a dream she was able to do the Magnetic Unruffle with her mother, and floods of tears as she told the story affirmed the validity of her inner healing. In a very different vein, a young participant dreamed the whole earth was on fire with pollution and chaos. In her despair, she began to smooth out the earth's energy field and to get some relief from the internal tension. She also joined an environmental awareness group after the dream.

## Activating the Three Injunctions

As mentioned, all inner explorative work must be done with care and respect. Brugh Joy (1979, pp. 60–61) tells the story of a very intuitive woman who was seeking self-understanding and heard a voice giving three specific instructions for her development. The three instructions appear as basic rules for operating in the self-exploratory, intrapersonal dimension: (1) Make no comparisons. (2) Make no judgments. (3) Delete your need to understand.

In a culture where achievement is highly valued, comparisons seem essential, and we are constantly trying to meet our own or others' high expectations. Judgments keep us locked in a prison of predictable patterns with little opportunity for new ideas or opening to others. The need to understand binds us into patterns of trying to analyze and figure out everything allowing little room for accepting and enjoying the mystery of life.

Comparisons, judgments, and overanalysis can be the basis of a workaholic lifestyle or an obsessive-compulsive personality pattern. They can drive us to stress-related disease and premature death. To counteract these possibilities, working with the three injunctions gives us a chance to break out of barriers. The following exercises can be used to break your unwanted thinking patterns until new ones become natural and automatic.

EXERCISE

## TO DECREASE COMPARISONS

1.  Ask your inner self to help you to be aware each time you make a comparison. The comparisons may be between yourself and others (Joe is smarter/dumber than I am) or between other people (Mary's is better/worse than Alice's).

2.  At the end of the day, in your journal write down the approximate number of these useless comparisons.

3.  After a while, you may wish to set your intent to change these unnecessary thought patterns. You can catch yourself midsentence or midthought and reprogram the thought.

4.  Work throughout the day with your intent to be less comparing and to become more accepting of things as they present themselves.

Deleting the need to understand means to drop *your* need to analyze things that are beyond comprehension. It certainly does not mean leaving your inquisitive nature or knowledge base behind. As we move in the path of learning about the deeper self, we often experience a coming together of unusual events, *synchronicities* as Jung called them, that suggest we are being led in a mysterious way. For instance, many students report finding information about an upcoming class just when they had received an unexpected check in the mail. Trying to figure out events like these could slow down the flow of life and take away the fun of enjoying the unexplainable. In extremes, we see persons with "paralysis of analysis," unable to move with spontaneity because everything has to be understood or planned on the mental level. In working to diminish your need for constant mental comprehension, you may want to note unusual events and trends that seem to be unfolding in your life.

## Creative Self-Expression

Another way to connect with one's inner resources is through creative self-expression. Since our goal is learning about the subconscious levels within, no artistic skill is needed here. Rather, use whatever medium is most suitable to express parts of yourself that might otherwise remain hidden. The secret, as always, is in centering first and remaining free of all judgmental or limiting thoughts (Seaton, 2001).

***Mandala Drawing***   Mandala drawing is an age-old technique in which one works with a circle on paper and allows the circle to fill either from the inside to the outer edges or from the outer rim to the middle. This is an example of a simple focusing device; you can use crayon, colored pencils, or pastels. As your interest progresses, you may enjoy the research that has been done utilizing mandala drawing as a form of art therapy (Kellogg, 1977) and luminous symbols for healing (Cornell, 1994).

***Object Arrangements***   Another easy way to connect with the inner being is through object arrangements. We often spontaneously gather up objects that have special meaning to us and create a place in the home for this collection. Doing this intentionally with the idea of making a meditation space could be one way of connecting safely with your inner being. This way of focusing can become highly therapeutic when, for instance, we assemble all the symbols evoking the memory of a friend to celebrate an event or to assist with grief work (Kazanis & Hover-Kramer, 1990).

***Creative Play***   Whatever the medium or the structure, let this be a time of flowing with your tools, feeling the movement of the inner rhythm and appreciating the results, however crude they may be. Jung regularly allowed an hour a day for sand play in his busy schedule, building cities, castles, and mandalas to have private, personal communication time that gave him immense satisfaction. Since then, whole schools of sand play techniques have evolved to utilize this delightful medium. Singing, dancing, or simply moving to music are other ways of playing without any particular intent other than self-discovery. The goal in creative play is to learn to trust the inner knowing and to recapture the spontaneity and joy that we knew as children.

## Meeting the Shadow

Self-knowledge means facing all parts of ourselves, even the parts we do not like. The shadow side of the personality is the designated bearer of the unknown and can be highly destructive if we ignore it. Notice, for example, how much easier it is to blame or shift feelings to someone else than to actually own the unpleasant parts of ourselves. Our conscious mental mechanisms are actually designed to suppress what is unpleasant as a self-protective mechanism and, often, vitally important. Just as we have a blind spot in driving that can cause accidents unless we learn to compensate, so we must learn to track this shadowy side of ourselves and learn its lessons.

A helpful way to begin tracking the shadow is to note the persons we dislike in an irrational way. Ask yourself what quality is most despicable about this person and how this might relate to something within yourself. For example, a practitioner found himself despising a certain client who was dependent and whiny. Instead of judging or withdrawing from the client, he asked what he could learn from the situation. In looking hard at his own hidden dependency needs, the healer was able to reconcile opposites within himself and see the client with more compassion.

***Projection*** When the shadow side is not confronted, we are likely to project our own uncomfortable feelings onto another. In the healing process, this countertransference, as it is known in the psychological literature, is a severe limitation to the therapeutic alliance. Energetically, the flow of unlimited potential from the universal through the healer is blocked. We may label a client as "difficult" or "unresponsive" when, in fact, *we* may be the persons who are unresponsive to significant client clues because of our own blind spots.

Worse, of course, is the projection of our unwanted parts onto a whole group of people. History abounds with examples. The Puritans of New England, for instance, liked things to be nice and tidy. "They feared swarthy Indians, probably were suspicious of dark-feathered turkeys, and walked uneasily in the pitchy pine woods of Massachusetts. For women they advised stockings, hoods, obedience, and silence. Hatred of the Yin (feminine) side of the circle begins as a small thread in the first American cloth. Hatred of Yin at the start gave New England a fierce energy; but three hundred years later, the same hatred drains people and leads to some sort of spiritual death" (Bly, 1988, p. 11).

These words recapture for us the power of the unconscious forces to evoke fear and projection when something is not understood. Thousands of healers, mostly women, who attuned to the mysteries of nature at a time when their cultures were overly rational, were burned as witches in the not too distant past.

As we learn about the personal shadow, we can also understand these mass projections. Although there may be no formal witch hunts today, there are hundreds of ways that the intuitive can be discounted and flattened. Since the reconciliation of our internal opposites is primary, we always begin by addressing the personal issues. From this daily work of self-awareness can come an attitude of inner harmony and peacefulness that allows us to face more public discounts or distractions with relative ease and nondefensiveness, without projection "hooks" as objecionable behaviors for others to latch onto. Reclaiming the shadow and integrating it allows us to acknowledge the unpleasant parts of ourselves but also to let our true selves emerge (Zweig & Abrams, 1991).

## OPENING TO THE TRANSPERSONAL PERSPECTIVE

The word *transpersonal* refers to the dimension of human consciousness that is greater than the personal, a *meta-* or *super*personal awareness. This connection with the dimension greater than the individual self is part of the spiritual journey that begins as we ask deeply about the meaning of life and death. This questing is quite distinct from a religious perspective that encompasses a set of specific beliefs and social forms of expression. Instead, the transpersonal refers to a world-view, an attitude, a process of self-discovery, and an expansion beyond personal pain or distress (Potter & Zniewski, 2000).

Currently, many therapists, counselors, and helping professionals are exploring the spiritual dimension as they look at resolving the many distortions and ills of our society. Throughout, the new textbook *Holistic Nursing* (Dossey et al., 2000), the spiritual dimension is explored as the heart of human caring and healing. The American Holistic Nurses' Association is a focal point for health caregivers who seek spiritual awareness, and the Association for Transpersonal Psychology provides many resources and publications for psychotherapists.

## Use with Self-Healing Techniques

The perspective that allows us to see ourselves as spiritual beings having temporary human experiences lifts and transforms our dilemmas and permits a wider dimension of self-healing to take place (Hover-Kramer, 1989). In her study of 35 caregivers, a nursing researcher found that working with the transpersonal, and allowing oneself to see a bigger picture, created a sense of meaning in difficult situations. Burnout among caregivers was significantly reduced when they moved beyond feelings of loss and devastation by evoking their connections with the Higher Self and a sense of meaning. "What emerged from the interviews as an over-riding theme of caring was the experience of spiritual transcendence. Spiritual transcendence was defined as experiencing oneself in relationship as a part of a force greater than oneself. This spiritual transcendence experience was critical not only in terms of the nurses' satisfaction with caring, but also as an explanation of the paradox of distance and closeness . . ." (Montgomery, 1991, p. 36).

As the traditions of self-healing through Alcoholics Anonymous and the related 12-step programs bear out (Mikluscak-Cooper & Miller, 1991; Small, 1991), problems are never solved at the level at which they were created. With our understanding of energy, we know that we vibrate to the same frequency as that to which we give primary attention. When we are bogged down in ordinary consciousness ruminating about an issue, we are vibrating at the energetic frequency of the problem. When we allow our perspective to shift, to attend to the Universal Will for the situation, we lift our vibrational frequency, just as a musician can raise a mood by going higher. The following exercise allows you to be aware of a problem and to let it change by looking at it with a different perspective, a different level of consciousness.

EXERCISE

## MOVING TO THE TRANSPERSONAL PERSPECTIVE

1.  Be aware of a problem that holds tension for you at this time. Allow yourself to look at the problem through your own eyes.

2.  Now, see the same problem through the eyes of someone who disagrees with you.

3.  Note the impasse this creates.

4.  Using your skills of centering and focused meditation, lift higher. Imagine you are looking at the whole thing from above, from an eagle's point of view, or how Higher Power as you understand it might see the issue.

5.  See someone you highly respect, Buddha or Jesus or Mary, handling the situation. Note how this person can see both sides of an issue while caring about you.

6.  Bring this awareness to the present situation, applying your new insight with compassion for yourself and the others involved.

Being in touch with our spirituality is not only uplifting but may indeed be life-saving when we think of the tremendous price our culture is currently paying through stress-related illnesses and burnout. "Humans have a profound need for transpersonal experiences and for states in which they transcend individual identities to feel their place in the large role that is timeless" (Grof & Bennett, 1992, p. 116). Apparently, this is part of our human development: to go beyond our ego selves, to evolve, and stretch to the farther reaches of our human natures.

## SUMMARY

We have attempted to outline some of the ways you might begin your personal quest for inner development. There are many paths, such as journal writing, dream work, paying attention to our inner dialogue, expressing creatively, meeting the shadow, and opening to the transpersonal perspective. Your work as an HT practitioner requires full awareness of yourself so that you can genuinely attune to others. The desire to help is the beginning, then, of a lifelong journey of self-discovery and increasing intrapersonal richness. It is a quest that is highly rewarding in facilitating your connection with others.

# REFERENCES

Bly, R. (1988). *A little book on the human shadow*. San Francisco: Harper and Row.

Cappachione, L. (1991). *The picture of health*. Santa Monica, CA: Hay House.

Cornell, J. (1994). *Mandala: Luminous symbols for healing*. Wheaton, IL: Quest Books.

Dossey, B., Frisch, N., Forker, J. & Levin, J. (1998). Evolving a blueprint for certification: Inventory of professional activities and knowledge of a holistic nurse. *Journal of Holistic Nursing, 16*, 33–56.

Dossey, B., Keegan, L. & Guzzetta, C. (2000). *Holistic nursing*. 3rd Ed., Gaithersburg, MD: Aspen Publishers.

Grof, S., & Bennett, H. Z. (1992). *The holotropic mind*. San Francisco: Harper and Row.

Hover-Kramer, D. (1989). Creating a context for self-healing: The transpersonal perspective. *Holistic Nursing Practice, 2*, 3.

Johnson, R. (1986). *Inner work*. San Francisco: Harper and Row.

Joy, B. (1979). *Joy's way*. Los Angeles: J. P. Tarcher, Inc.

Jung, C. G. (1974). *Dreams*. Princeton, NJ: Bollingen Series.

Kazanis, B., & Hover-Kramer, D. (1990). Object arrangement. *Beginnings, 10*, 4.

Keegan, L. & Dossey, B. (1998). *Profiles of nurse healers*. Albany, NY: Delmar.

Kellogg, J., MacRae, M., Bonny, H., & Di Leo, F. (1977). The use of the mandala in psychiatric evaluation and treatment. *American Journal of Art Therapy, 7*, 123–134.

Khan, P. V. I. (1982). *Introducing spirituality into counseling and therapy*. Lebanon Springs, NY: Omega Press.

Mikluscak-Cooper, C., & Miller, E. (1991). *Living in hope*. Berkeley, CA: Celestial Arts.

Montgomery, C. (1991). The caregiving relationships, paradoxical and transcendent aspects. *Journal of Transpersonal Psychology, 12*, 3.

Potter, M. L. & Zauszniewski, J. A. (Dec., 2000). Spirituality, resourcefulness and arthritis impact on health perception of elders with rheumatoid arthritis. *Journal of Holistic Nursing 18* (4), 311–331.

Progoff, I. (1975). *At a journal workshop*. New York: Dialogue House.

Rainer, T. (1978). *The new diary*. Los Angeles: J. P. Tarcher, Inc.

Rew, L. (June, 2000). Acknowledging intuition in clinical decision making. *Journal of Holistic Nursing 18* (2), 94–108.

Seaton, J. (2001). *Artlife*. 12 tape series. Boulder, CO: Sounds True.

Slater, V., Maloney, J., Krau, S., & Eckert, C. (1999). Journey to Holism. *Journal of Holistic Nursing, 17* (4), 365–383.

Small, J. (1991). *Awakening in time*. New York: Bantam Books.

Thurston, M. (1978). *How to interpret your dreams*. Virginia Beach, VA: A.R.E. Press.

Zweig, C. & Abrams, J., Eds. (1991). *Meeting the shadow*. New York: G. P. Putnam's Sons.

# CHAPTER 19

# Conclusion—Opening to the Next Decade of Healing Touch

*"At our deepest level we are spirit
Touching the world of higher consciousness
And reaching out to the heartbeat of humanity."*

—Dorothea Hover-Kramer

## INTRODUCTION

As we come to the conclusion of this exploration of Healing Touch, we are open and filled with wonder and curiosity about developments within the next decade. The whole framework of health care seems to be rapidly shifting as new understandings of healing, relationship with our environments, and the transpersonal dimension evolve. These transformations are part of a vast paradigm change, one that began with the holistic medical and nursing organizations, developed more fully with increasing emphasis on wellness and complementary modalities, and is coming to fruition in an explosion of research and rapidly expanding information in all the major sciences.

From the perspective of health and healing, we are living in the most exciting of times. Let us explore a few of the trends that are emerging in the 21st century and that will continue to resonate in healing practices in the years to come.

## CONTINUING EXPANSION OF COMPLEMENTARY MODALITIES

In 1992 the first national office to study alternative medicine (OAM) opened in the National Institutes of Health (NIH). In 2000 this office has developed into the National Center for Complementary and Alternative Medicine (NCCAM), a fully funded, separate arm of the NIH (Stokstad, 2000). The over $80 million budget will foster research in such complementary modalities as acupuncture and herbal treatments for depression and arthritis. A new investigation of "frontier medicine" has been funded to study therapies for which there are no known biological mechanisms, such as magnets, energy healing, and homeopathy.

Another milestone is the establishment of the White House Commission on Complementary and Alternative Medicine in July, 2000. Headed by James S. Gordon, MD, a well-known leader in mind/body modalities, it will generate a profound impact on medical practice in the 21st century, comparable to the impact of the Flexner report and its impact on medical practice in the 20th century. Dr. Gordon (2000) writes, "At the beginning of the 21st century, Congress and the president are asking a commission of conventional physicians and researchers, complementary and alternative medicine pioneers, citizen advocates, and business people—men and women of many colors and ethnic backgrounds—to design a new blueprint for a new medicine that is both scientific and inclusive."

Clinics and research centers, like the Center for Integrative Medicine at the prestigious Scripps Hospitals in San Diego, CA, are developing nationwide. In conjunction with the Ornish cardiology center at Scripps, cardiologist Dr. Mimi Guaneri and her nurse colleague Rauni King are investigating the effects of energy healing. As Ms. King is a well-established Healing Touch practitioner and instructor, it is possible that this will be one of the areas chosen for one of the "frontier medicine" investigations (personal communication, Dr. Phyllis Mabbett, program administrator, May, 2001).

Nationally, the work of Barbara and Larry Dossey and their many colleagues is bringing a whole new awareness of the meaning of holism. Nursing's own Barbara Dossey has spearheaded the development of a nationwide holistic nursing curriculum and published the third edition of the classic *Holistic Nursing* text (Dossey et al., 2000). In medicine and alternative therapies, Larry Dossey, MD, continues to publish the noted peer-reviewed journal *Alternative Therapies in Health and Medicine*, now in its sixth year. The November 2000 issue, for instance, has seven articles reporting on complementary modalities, in addition to the news about the White House Commission quoted above. With each issue, updates of the activities of NCCAM and the White House Commission are given (Muscat, 2001). New ways of seeing the world of health care surround us professionally and in the media and such changes will undoubtedly continue to accelerate.

# INCREASING STUDIES OF CONSCIOUSNESS AND ENERGY

Research on human consciousness, as yet in early stages, is yielding fascinating results about the impact of intent on matter (Radin, Rebman and Cross, 1996). Centers for the study of consciousness are developing in conjunction with major universities, including the University of Nevada, Princeton University, and the University of Arizona in Tuscon.

Specific research into the nature of human energy fields and nonlocal communication is continuing to develop in centers like the Menninger Institute, in Topeka, KS, and the California Institute of Human Sciences in Encinitas, CA. Under the leadership of chief researcher Dr. Gaetan Chevalier, the latter institute has developed a computerized tool for measuring meridians to assist in diagnosis, as well as doing experimental work in assessing chakras and biofields (personal communication, April, 2001). It is quite possible that standardized measures of the human vibrational matrix will replace more invasive diagnostic tools within the next ten years (Gerber, 2001).

# ACCEPTANCE OF SPIRITUALITY AS CENTRAL TO HEALING

In recent years, spirituality has "come out of the closet" as an integral aspect of healing practice. A flood of articles and literature reviews, conferences, and seminars place care of the human spirit at the heart of effective health care (Burkhardt, 1994; Coberly & Shapiro, 1998; Sumner, 1998; McGee, 2000). In just the past few years, it has become acceptable to discuss spiritual concerns just as one would address the psychosocial needs of the client, and to do so within a framework of caring without judgment or expectation of any particular belief system. Ecospirituality, a holistic combining of spiritual and environmental concerns, is developing as a new manifestation and expression of interest in healing our planet and all its citizens. Healing ceremonies are a part of many hospital settings, and some facilities even have developed ways of spiritually nurturing their personnel. In Healing Touch, advanced practitioners connect with their clients in profoundly touching and deeply spiritual ways.

## The Story of Sallie, the Cat Lady

A year ago I received three desperate calls from the adult children of a local artist whom I will call Sallie. Each of them insisted that my visiting her and giving a Healing Touch session would somehow save her life, as neither radiation nor chemotherapy had affected her galloping intestinal cancer. As it happened, I was in her area the next week and made a rare home visit. As I rang the doorbell, a distinguished large brown dog came to the door and signaled that I should enter. With some hesitancy I did, to find that Buzz, the dog, was master of a herd of grown cats, 43 to be exact. They were strays whom Sallie had retrieved from "death row" at the local Humane Society shelter over the period of several years.

Sallie greeted me from the couch. She was emaciated, weighing only 65 pounds. Her face was gray. As three cats surrounded her with snuggles, I gently began the Magnetic Unruffle, finding some difficulty in maneuvering around a boisterous young tomcat. Mostly, I worked hard to stay centered in this complicated environment. And, although I seldom use directional prayer, I prayed that she might live if possible for the sake of these many little furry ones.

I never heard from the adult children or from Sallie. I assumed she had passed on because of her condition. Just this month I received a call. Sallie sounded strong and healthy and said she would like to come to my office for another Healing Touch session. It was a treat to see the slim, tall woman with rosy cheeks enter my door. More radiation given after my session seemed to have destroyed the cancer but unfortunately it also injured her hip and she had received a hip replacement. Nonetheless, Sallie was healthy and able to minister to her "cat family."

Her problem now was "loss of soul;" somewhere between the surgeries and challenging year Sallie lost her sense of connection with her Higher Power. She said, "I pray but nothing seems to happen." She was unable to return to her art work; something had run dry. When I pointed out that I thought she was dying a year earlier and now she was alive and well, she became thoughtful. "Maybe my prayers have been answered but I don't feel any connection with God." She seemed touched when I mentioned I had prayed for her.

Together, we asked that this healing session be for Sallie's highest good. After I cleared her field for about ten minutes, I began the Full Body Connection. I felt a marked chill in the room although it was a warm day. From then on, I followed my hands, which seemed to be guided in rhythms I did not fully understand. At the end of the session, I asked Sallie to share her personal experience. She reported that she held one thought, "Please come and let me receive your help." After ten minutes of relaxing, Sallie saw the room fill with light, she felt her angels around her in a most tangible way. She cried softly as she described her sense of oneness with the Infinite. For the first time since we met, Sallie smiled. She said she felt a sense of great peace and confidence. She was ready to resume artistic expression again. And her hip no longer hurt.

In the realm of traditional medical, counseling, or nursing practice there is no context for these kinds of experiences. In the realm of our expanding definitions of healing and caring encounters through practices like Healing Touch, such stories are a frequent occurrence. Many of our experienced practitioners could recount similar, fascinating stories. Accessing the spiritual dimension is ultimately the most powerful healing of human woundedness, as it resonates throughout the human energy field bringing new information to the mental, emotional, and physical dimensions.

# ONGOING EXPLORATIONS

The story of Healing Touch, begun just eleven years ago, continues to develop. As we practice the techniques, we will learn new approaches from the interactions with our clients. As we center ourselves, we will open to new levels of self-awareness. As we encounter difficulties, we will ask many more questions. As we observe the phenomena around us, we will develop new theories about healing. We as caregivers are part of an ongoing, evolutionary process that opens to full human potential.

We close with a healing meditation:

> In the space between the last thought
> And a future image
> Rests the moment,
> The Now of the timeless
> Spaceless present.
> In the instant of my intent
> And your reaching out for peace
> Comes the healing—
> Interacting fields
> Chakras opening
> Energies balancing
> Alignment to the Eternal Light.

# REFERENCES

Burkhardt, M. A. (1994). Becoming and connecting: Elements of spirituality for women. *Holistic Nursing Practice, 8* (4), 12–21.

Coberly, M. & Shapiro, S. I. (1998). A transpersonal approach to care of the dying. *Journal of Transpersonal Psychology, 30* (1), 1–38.

Dossey, B., Keegan, L., & Guzetta, C. F. (Eds.) (2000). *Holistic nursing.* Gaithersburg, MD: Aspen Publishing.

Gerber, R. (2001). *Vibrational medicine.* Rochester, VT: Bear & Co.

Gordon, J. S. (Nov., 2000). The White House Commission and the future of healthcare. *Alternative Therapies, 6* (6), 26–28.

Lincoln, V. (Sept., 2000). Ecospirituality: A pattern that connects. *Journal of Holistic Nursing, 18* (3), 227–243.

McGee, E. M. (March, 2000). AA and nursing: Lessons in holism and spiritual care. *Journal of Holistic Nursing, 18* (1), 11–26.

Muscat, M. (March, 2001). Strauss gives state of the center. *Alternative Therapies, 7* (2), 23–26.

Radin, D. I., Rebman, J. M., & Cross, M. P. (1996). Anomalous organization of random events by group consciousness: Two exploratory experiments. *Journal of Scientific Exploration, 10* (1), 143–168.

Stokstad, E. (June 2, 2000). Stephen Straus's impossible job. *Science, 288,* 1568–1570.

Sumner, C. H. (1998). Recognizing and responding to spiritual distress. *American Journal of Nursing, 98* (1), 26–31.

# Appendices

# APPENDIX A

# Glossary

**Aura:** Metaphysical term for the human energy field, or biofield.

**Balancing:** Term used to describe the realignment of the biofield to its natural, highest vibrational function and potentials.

**Biofield:** A scientific term for the vibrational emanations that surround and extend beyond the human body, as measured by SQUID (Superconducting Quantum Interference Device) and demonstrated through the mechanism of Kirlian photography.

**Centering:** The process of focusing one's attention and intention to be fully responsive and present to one's client, setting aside personal issues and outcome expectations.

**Chakra:** Sanskrit word meaning spinning wheel, used to name the human energy centers, or vortices. Also known as centers of consciousness, due to the psychological and developmental properties of each center.

**Ch'i:** (preferred spelling is *Qi* and is pronounced "chee.") Chinese term for energy or vital life force that acts as nourishing subtle flow through the chakras, the meridians, and the biofield. Also called *prana, ki,* or *spiritus.*

**Clearing:** The facilitator's hand movements above the biofield that facilitate the release of energy blockage. Synonymous with releasing, letting go, smoothing, or unruffling of the biofield.

**Energy Blockage:** A general term that refers to the interruption or constriction of the natural flow patterns in the human vibrational matrix. May refer to a closed or diminished chakra, asymmetry in the biofield, or non-polarity and reversal in the meridian flows.

**Energy Center:** Same as chakra, a specific center of consciousness in the human vibrational matrix that allows inflow of *Qi* to the human organism from the Universal Energy Field, and outflow of excessive *Qi* from the human body-mind.

**Energy Healing:** Broad term used to describe interventions that address the releasing of energetic blockage or imbalance, followed by repatterning, balancing, and aligning of the human vibrational matrix to higher levels of functioning.

**Focusing:** The holding of positive intent in relation to a specific aspect of the biofield or a chakra to allow for repatterning, balancing, and modulation of energy. This focusing or holding of intent can be assisted by placing the hands over the area and is generally done after clearing maneuvers.

**241**

**Grounding:** Connecting to the earth and earth's energy field to calm the mind and balance the entire energy system.

**Healing:** The ongoing evolution toward ever higher levels of functioning in the multidimensional human being.

**Human Energy System:** The entire interactive dynamic of human subtle energies consisting of the chakras, the multidimensional field, the meridians, and their acupoints; the human vibrational matrix of subtle energy.

**Intention:** Holding one's inner awareness and focus to accomplish a specific task or activity; being fully present in the moment.

**Modulation of Energy:** Process of holding hands over a specific area to assist in restoring balance, often done after clearing areas of blockage or disruptions in the flow of *Qi*.

**Psychoenergetic Healing:** A form of healing practice that interrelates psychological insights with understanding of the human vibrational matrix.

**Spiritual:** As differentiated from any specific religious belief or practice, this word describes each person's unique connection to some quality that is greater than the personal self. Practices to enhance spiritual awareness may include being still, meditating, praying, breathing purposefully, grounding to the earth, setting intent, journaling, crafting, creating, listening carefully, and learning to trust intuition.

**Transpersonal:** Term coined by Drs. Abraham Maslow, Anthony Sutich, and Stanislav Grof, founders of the Association for Transpersonal Psychology, to describe the psychological realm beyond the purely personal, reaching to the wider, spiritual dimension of human experience.

**Universal Energy Field:** Term to describe the infinite resource of unlimited energy that surrounds and interpenetrates all aspects of the Universe.

**Unruffling:** Term coined by Dr. Dolores Krieger to suggest the clearing or smoothing of a ruffled, disturbed area in the biofield.

# Resources for
# Further Information

**Healing Touch (HT)**
Colorado Center for HT (CCHT)
Administrative information, course schedules, newsletter, & local network information
12477 W. Cedar Dr., Suite 206, Lakewood, CO, 80228
Tel. 303-989-0581; FAX 303-985-9702
Email—ccheal@aol.com
Website—www.healingtouch.net

**Healing Touch International (HTI)**
Certification program information, international programs
12477 W. Cedar Drive, Suite 202, Lakewood, CO, 80228
Tel. 303-989-7982; FAX 303-980-8683
Email—HTheal@aol.com

**Therapeutic Touch (TT)**
Nurse Healers—Professional Associates, Inc. (NH—PAI)
760 South Highland Dr., Suite 429
Salt Lake City, UT 84106
Tel. 801-942-5900
Email—RMGOOD@worldnet.att.net
Website—www.therapeutictouch.org

**Holistic Nursing**
American Holistic Nurses' Association (AHNA)
PO Box 2130
Flagstaff, AZ 86003-2130
Tel. 800-526-AHNA; FAX 520-526-2752
Email—AHNA-Flag@Flaglink.com
Website—ahna.org

**Subtle Energy Medicine**
International Society for the Study of Subtle Energies/Energy Medicine
(ISSSEEM)
356 Golden Circle
Golden, CO 80403
Tel. 303-278-2228

**Energy Psychology**
Association for Comprehensive Energy Psychology (ACEP)
c/o Dr. Dorothea Hover-Kramer
12307 Oak Knoll Rd., Suite B
Poway, CA, 92064
Tel. 656-748-5963; FAX 858-748-3119
Emails—DRGrudermeyer@willingness.com; Dorotheah@aol.com
website—www.energypsych.org

# The Certification Process to Become a Certified Healing Touch Practitioner

(Presented with acknowledgement of the support of the American Holistic Nurses' Association.)

The purpose for awarding certification as a Healing Touch Practitioner is to document the collected experiences of the individual, to acknowledge competent and experienced practice based on an established educational program, to identify and acknowledge the new professional, and to communicate with the public by recognizing this educational preparation. The certificate ensures that the participant in the program has achieved a level of skill and personal growth that is comparable to others at the same level of expertise.

The following criteria must be met for certification:

1. Completion of all coursework for the Healing Touch Practitioner: Level I, Level II-A, Level II-B, Level III-A, Level III-B.

2. Evidence of receiving ten different healing modalities with professionals; evidence of giving 100 Healing Touch sessions of which the ten best are documented in paragraph form.

3. Development of a professional profile notebook which includes a comprehensive resume, articles written by or about the individual, detailed listing of conferences and educational experiences related to professional practice.

4. Presentation of brief resume of all education, licenses, and experience, including Healing Touch workshops, dates, places, and instructors.

5. Mentorship with a certified Healing Touch practitioner for one year or more, documented by a written evaluation of the experience by the mentor and a self-report from the individual.

6. Evidence of ongoing reading and related educational experiences described in paragraph form (15–20 books, tapes studied, conferences attended, etc.).

7. Development of a descriptive case study of work in depth with one client to demonstrate a minimum of 3–5 sessions including intake, assessment, treatment planning, implementation, evaluation, referrals, and discharge planning.

8. A self-study describing personal development throughout the educational program, plans for continued personal and spiritual growth, development of the practice of Healing Touch in the community and in the world as a whole.

For further information about Healing Touch Certification, please contact:

Healing Touch International, Inc.
12477 W. Cedar Dr. Suite 202
Lakewood, CO 80228

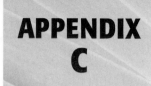

# APPENDIX C

# Sample Informed Consent

I understand that Healing Touch is a complementary modality that in no way substitutes for appropriate medical intervention, body therapy, or psychotherapy. I also understand that my practitioner will make suggestions for my self-care and referrals based on wide experience.

I recognize that there is a close working partnership between me and my practitioner that requires me to share my ideas, perceptions, and opinions readily. In this manner any misunderstandings can be cleared up immediately.

I further understand that there are numerous benefits possible through Healing Touch, such as diminished pain sensation, increased relaxation, relief from anxiety, and enhanced sense of well-being. These effects may vary depending on each individual's response patterns. Although there are no known harmful effects from this type of intervention, I hold my practitioner harmless from any possible effects that may cause temporary discomfort and agree to take full responsibility for my self-care and personal development.

Signed _____

Printed Name _____

Date _____

# Sample Intake Sheet

**Date**

**Identifying Data**

| | |
|---|---|
| Name _____ | Telephone # _____ |
| Address _____ | Zip _____ |
| Profession _____ | |
| Referred by _____ | Date of birth _____ |

**Physical Status**
    Presenting symptoms
    Current medications
    Pertinent medical history, including surgeries

**Emotional Status**
    Current stress in personal life
    Current stress in professional life
    Current sources of pleasure
    Client rating of emotional health

**Mental Status**
    Predominant thought patterns
    Meditation experience
    Effectiveness of inner practices
    Client rating of mental health

**Spiritual Awareness**
    Client sense of connection to higher power
    Spiritual practices used by client
    Effectiveness of spiritual practices

**Energetic Assessment**
    Areas of energy field disturbance/imbalance
    Condition of the major chakras
    Intuitive perceptions of practitioner

# INDEX